Veterinary Treatment of Pigs

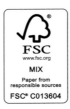

I would like to dedicate this book to Alec Dawson MRCVS who was my guide and mentor when I first returned to general practice in the UK in 1975. Although he was in his late sixties he always kept updated and was always prepared to give helpful, friendly advice.

I had only been working for him for 4 weeks when he suggested that my knowledge of pig medicine was rather limited. He showed me an advertisement for a two-day pig medicine course advertised in the *Veterinary Record*. I duly attended at the practice expense. That course and his knowledge were the foundation of my pig practice. I will always remember him with gratitude.

Veterinary Treatment of Pigs

Graham R. Duncanson

Westover Veterinary Centre, UK

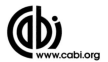
www.cabi.org

CABI is a trading name of CAB International

CABI	CABI
Nosworthy Way	38 Chauncey Street
Wallingford	Suite 1002
Oxfordshire OX10 8DE	Boston, MA 02111
UK	USA
Tel: +44 (0)1491 832111	Tel: +1 800 552 3083 (toll free)
Fax: +44 (0)1491 833508	Tel: +1 (0)617 395 4051
E-mail: info@cabi.org	E-mail: cabi-nao@cabi.org
Website: www.cabi.org	

A catalogue record for this book is available from the British Library, London, UK.

Library of Congress Cataloging-in-Publication Data

Duncanson, Graham R., author.
Veterinary treatment of pigs / Graham R. Duncanson.
    p. ; cm.
  Includes bibliographical references and index.
  ISBN 978-1-78064-172-0 (alk. paper)
  I. C.A.B. International, issuing body. II. Title.
[DNLM: 1. Sus scrofa. 2. Swine Diseases. 3. Animal Husbandry. SF 971]

  SF996.5
  616.02'73--dc23

                       2013019853

ISBN-13: 978 1 78064 172 0

Commissioning editor: Sarah Hulbert
Editorial assistant: Alexandra Lainsbury
Production editor: Shankari Wilford

Typeset by SPi, Pondicherry, India
Printed and bound in the UK by CPI Group (UK) Ltd, Croydon, CR0 4YY.

Contents

Acknowledgements

I would like to acknowledge the considerable help I have obtained from reading two excellent textbooks while I was writing this book: *Pig Diseases* (8th edition) by D.J. Taylor (ISBN 0 9506932 7 8) and *Handbook of Pig Medicine* by Peter G.G. Jackson and Peter D. Cockcroft (ISBN 978 0 7020 2828 1). They have helped considerably to triangulate all the information.

I would also like to thank my editor Sarah Hulbert who has been a constant source of advice and encouragement.

Finally I would like to thank all my colleagues who have helped me with the pictures, particularly my daughter for all her patience on our numerous travels in search of information.

Abbreviations

AA	amino acid
ad lib	*ad libitum,* as much as desired
AGID	agar gel immunodiffusion
AI	artificial insemination
ALP	alkaline phosphatase
ASF	African swine fever
AST	aspartate aminotransferase
BHC	benzene hexachloride
BSE	bovine spongiform encephalopathy
CFT	complement fixation test
CK	creatine kinase
CNS	central nervous system
CSF	cerebrospinal fluid or classical swine fever
DEFRA	Department for Environment, Food and Rural Affairs
DON	deoxynivalenol
DVM	Divisional Veterinary Manager
EDTA	ethylene diamine tetra-acetic acid
ELISA	enzyme-linked immunosorbent assay
FAT	fluorescent antibody test
FEC	faecal egg count
FMD	foot and mouth disease
GA	general anaesthetic
GGT	γ-glutamyltransferase
GI	gastrointestinal
GLDH	glutamate dehydrogenase
GnRF/GnRH	gonadotrophin-releasing hormone
Hb	haemoglobin
IBR	inclusion body rhinitis
im	intramuscularly
ip	intraperitoneally
iv	intravenously
MCF	malignant catarrhal fever
MMA	mastitis, metritis, agalactia syndrome

NSAID	non-steroidal anti-inflammatory drug
OBF	Officially Brucellosis Free
OIE	Office International des Epizooties
Ov-HV2	ovine herpes type 2 virus
PCMV	porcine cytomegalovirus infection
PCR	polymerase chain reaction
PCV	packed cell volume
PCV-2	porcine circovirus type 2
PDNS	porcine dermatitis and nephropathy syndrome
PE	proliferative enteropathy
PEARS	porcine epidemic abortion and respiratory syndrome
PED	porcine epidemic diarrhoea
PGF$_{2\alpha}$	prostaglandin F$_{2\alpha}$
PHE	proliferative haemorrhagic enteropathy
PIA	porcine intestinal adenomatosis complex
PME	post-mortem examination
PMSG	pregnant mare serum gonadotrophin
PMWS	post-weaning multisystemic wasting syndrome
po	*per os*, orally
PPV	porcine parvovirus
PRRS	porcine reproductive and respiratory syndrome
PSS	porcine stress syndrome
RAPD PCR	random amplification of polymorphic DNA–PCR
RBC	red blood cell
RBPT	Rose Bengal plate test
RNA	ribonucleic acid
RT-PCR	reverse transcriptase PCR
SAC	South American camelid
sc	subcutaneously
SF	swine fever
SG	specific gravity
SIV	swine influenza virus
SMEDI	stillbirths, mummification, embryonic deaths and infertility
SOP	Standard Operating Procedure
SVD	swine vesicular disease
TAT	tetanus antiserum
TGE	transmissible gastroenteritis
TTV	torque teno virus
VO	Veterinary Officer
VTEC	verocytotoxigenic *Escherichia coli*
WBC	white blood cell
WFSI	weaning to fertile service interval
WOI	weaning to oestrus interval

1 Animal Husbandry

The Origins of the Domestic Pig

These are confused as the traditional view was that the pig was domesticated in Southeast Asia and then was brought westwards to Central Asia and on to Europe. There is some genetic evidence that domestication occurred also in Eastern Europe and there may well have been some crossing of early domestic pigs. Certainly the European wild boar (*Sus scrofu*) was involved in the 4th millennium BC in Europe (Fig. 1.1). Equally, there is evidence of domestication 9000 years ago in the Mekong Delta in Vietnam. By referencing the pig genome some authors (Groenen *et al.*, 2012) have discovered that there was a deep phylogenetic split between European and Asian wild boars around one million years ago, substantiating the hypothesis that pigs were independently domesticated in western Eurasia and East Asia. The pig has become part of the culture of Southeast Asia (Fig. 1.2).

The pig is a forest animal (Fig. 1.3). It does not lend itself to being driven like cattle, sheep and goats and so its domestication will have been delayed until man had a more sedentary existence.

Breeds of Pig

Aksai Black Pied

This large breed of pig with its distinctive black and white colouring originates from Kazakhstan.

Arapawa Island

These small pigs from New Zealand probably are descended from pigs allowed to become feral, having been released by Captain Cook. They are pigs with a light body, normally sandy with black spots. They do not have wattles.

Auckland Island Pig

This small breed of pig from the North Island of New Zealand is black or black and tan in colour.

Ba Xuyen

These pigs are derived from crossing Berkshire pigs and Chinese pigs from the Mekong Delta.

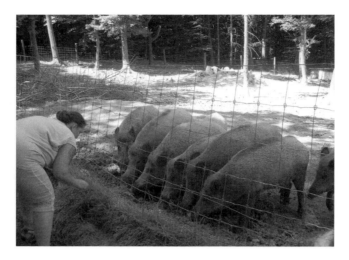

Fig. 1.1. Commercial wild boar in Austria.

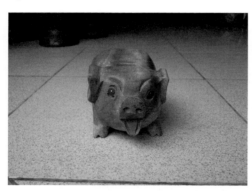

Fig. 1.2. A carved pig. Pigs have become part of the culture of South-east Asia.

They are a medium-sized pig with a very thickset body. They are mainly black with some white markings.

Bantu

The origins of this breed are obscure. They come from Southern Africa. They are a small medium-sized pig with an athletic build. They are mainly black or white with multiple black spots (Fig. 1.4).

Bazna

This large pig, which is black and white, originates from Romania.

Beijing Black

As the name suggests, this is a Chinese black pig of medium size (Fig. 1.5).

Belarus Black Pied

This black and white pig is similar to the Bazna but is normally larger.

Bentheim Black Pied

This very large black and white pig originates from Germany.

Berkshire

This large British pig is mainly black. It is not a rare breed as such but the numbers are now small. Small amounts of white on the pig are acceptable.

British Lop

This large white British pig has lop ears.

Bulgaria White

This is a large white pig with upright ears.

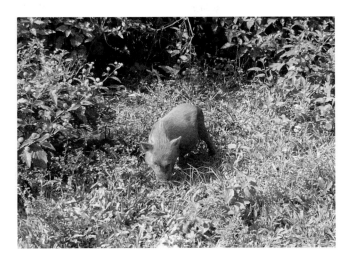

Fig. 1.3. Pigs are forest animals.

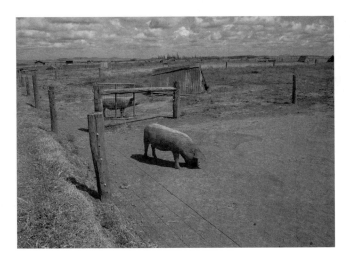

Fig. 1.4. A cross-bred Bantu pig.

Chato Murciano

These medium-sized pigs originate from Spain. They are black, white or black and white.

Danish Protest Pig

These very large pigs, as the name suggests, were bred in Denmark. They are red with a white saddle. They have lop ears.

Choctaw Hog

These very small black pigs originated in the USA.

Duroc

These large fecund pigs were bred in the USA. They are normally red but may be black.

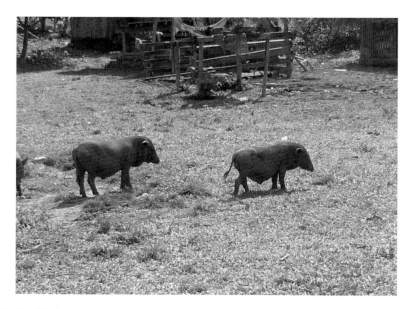

Fig. 1.5. Beijing Black weaners.

They have lop ears. There is Duroc blood found in many hybrids.

Forest Mountain

This is a large white pig which originated in Armenia.

Gascon

This is a large black pig with lop ears which originated in Gascony in France.

Gloucestershire Old Spot

This is a large, mainly white pig with large black spots. It has lop ears and originated in Gloucestershire in the UK. It was a rare breed but it has had resurgence in recent years (Fig. 1.6). It is much sought after by smallholders because of its quiet temperament. There is a niche market for its meat.

Guinea Hog

This medium-sized black pig has prick ears. It originated in the USA.

Hampshire

This is a medium-sized pig, with prick ears. It originated in Hampshire in the UK. It is normally a saddleback but some are all black. It is a quiet pig and is seen on smallholdings throughout the South of England.

Hereford

This breed of pig, which can be very large, is normally red and white. It originated in the USA.

Iberian

This medium-sized black pig originated in Spain. It has lop ears.

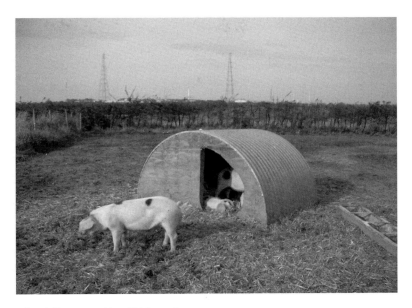

Fig. 1.6. Pure-bred Gloucestershire Old Spot pigs.

Jeju Black Pig

The name describes everything about this breed of pig. It is black and originated in Jeju-do in Korea. It is a small pig with lop ears.

Kakhetian

This black pig is small with prick ears. Grey and reddish brown pigs are also seen. It originated in Europe and is now only found in Georgia. The piglets have stripes which disappear on maturity.

Kemerovo

This is a small black pig with prick ears which originated in Kazakhstan.

Korea Native Pig

This is a medium-sized black pig with lop ears which is found in Korea.

Kunekune

These small pigs with long hair from New Zealand are very popular as pet pigs in the UK. They have several recognizable colours: red, black and white, cream, gold-tip, black, brown and tricoloured. They all have wattles called piri-piri (Fig. 1.7). They are friendly pigs and are ideal as a smallholder pig. As the gene pool in the UK is small, purchasers should beware of any inherited defects. They are often crossed with Vietnamese pigs to make 'house-pigs' (Fig. 1.8). They are also crossed with commercial hybrid pigs to make better carcasses for pig meat (Figure 1.9).

Lacombe

This is an old breed developed in Alberta in Canada from crossing Landrace and Berkshire pigs. It is a large breed, has lop ears and is normally black, but white animals are seen.

Landrace

There are now many separate breeds of Landrace pig, e.g. American, British, Danish, Dutch,

Finnish, French, German, Italian, Japanese, Norwegian and Swedish. They all originate from Scandinavia. They are a very important breed now used extensively in hybrids. They are a large white pig with lop ears, renowned for their length and limited back fat.

Large Black

This large English breed is all black with lop ears.

Large White

This large English breed is all white and has prick ears. It forms the basis of many hybrids

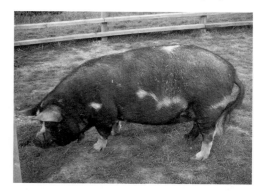

Fig. 1.7. A Kunekune pig. Note the wattles.

used in commercial pig production. It is particularly useful when crossed with a Landrace-type pig.

Latvian White

As the name suggests, this large white pig was developed in Latvia. It has prick ears.

Lithuanian White

This all white, large pig with prick ears was developed in Lithuania by crossing English Large White pigs with Lithuanian native pigs. These native pigs were either black and white or red and white.

Lincolnshire Curly-Coated

This large white pig, as the name suggests, has an abundant curly coat. It has prick ears and was developed in Lincolnshire.

Mangalitsa

This medium-sized pig with a large girth has lop ears. It can be red or tan or even partly black. It was developed in Hungary.

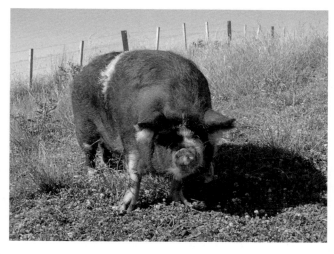

Fig. 1.8. A Kunekune pig crossed with a Vietnamese pig in New Zealand.

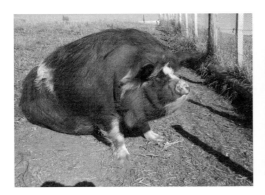

Fig. 1.9. A Kunekune pig crossed with a commercial hybrid pig.

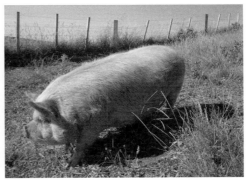

Fig. 1.10. A Middle White pig crossed with a Kunekune pig in New Zealand.

Meishan

This is a medium-sized pig with little hair and large folds of skin not only on its body but also on its head. It has lop ears and is pinky black in colour. It originated in China.

Middle White

Although in theory this breed of pig is smaller than a Large White pig, it is still categorized as a large pig. It is all white with prick ears. It has a very short snout. The breed was developed in Yorkshire in the UK. Middle White pigs are often crossed with Kunekune pigs to make pet pigs (Fig. 1.10).

Mukota

This small fat pig was developed in Zimbabwe to be resistant to the heat and tropical diseases. It is black with a short snout and lop ears.

Mulefoot

This is a very strange breed of pig which was developed in the USA from original stock from the Deep South. It is now a rare breed. It does not have a cloven hoof; hence its name, as its foot looks like that of a mule. The lack of a cloven hoof is in fact an inherited defect. The ethics of breeding these pigs must be questionable. It is normally all black but some have white spots.

Myrhorod

This is a medium-sized white pig with lop ears which was developed in the Ukraine.

North Caucasian

This is a hybrid pig bred from native pigs and imported Landrace blood in southern Russia and in Uzbekistan. It is normally a large white pig with lop ears.

North Siberian

This is a small curly-coated pig from northern Siberia. It has prick ears and is normally brown in colour. It manages to cope with the extremely harsh climate.

Ossabaw Island

This small pig is derived from feral pigs bred on Ossabaw Island which lies in the Atlantic Ocean off Georgia in the USA. It has prick ears and is normally black or spotted.

Oxford Sandy and Black

These are an old breed of medium-sized pigs which are almost considered a rare bred in the UK. They are a sandy colour with large black spots. They have lop ears.

Pietrain

These middle-sized pigs originated in Belgium and form a part of modern European hybrid commercial pigs. They are white in colour with large grey spots. They have prick ears. They are renowned for their large muscle to bone and fat ratio.

Red Wattle

This is a very large pig from the USA. It is red in colour and has lop ears.

Saddleback

There are now many separate breeds of Saddleback, e.g. the Angeln from Germany, the British Saddleback, the Essex and the Wessex. They are a large pig, mainly black with a white band around their girth. They have lop ears.

Semirechye

This middle-sized pig breed originated in Kazakhstan. It is usually used as a crossing sire for breeding hybrid gilts. It is black in colour with prick ears.

Siberian Black Pied

This small hairy pig comes from Siberia. It is black and white with prick ears.

Small Black

This small black pig from the UK with lop ears is now a rare breed. Traditionally it was a smallholder or backyard pig.

Small White

This small white pig from the UK has prick ears and is rare. It is still used to breed hybrids for commercial pig production. It has been selectively bred from so that its offspring are very small. These are then marketed as 'mini pigs'. They are also called 'designer pigs'. Purchasers should be aware that often they can grow into quite large pigs.

Swabian-Hall

This medium-sized pig from Germany is white with large black patches. It has lop ears and a long back. It is ideal as a bacon-producing pig.

Taihu Pig

This small black pig from China has prick ears and a long snout.

Tamworth

This large red pig from the UK is once again gaining in popularity as a smallholder pig supplying a niche pork market. It is a docile pig with prick ears. It is not a rare breed (Fig. 1.11).

Tsivilsk

This small all white pig with prick ears originated in Russia.

Turopolje

This medium-sized white black-spotted pig originated in Croatia and is considered by many to be one of the oldest pig breeds in Europe. Its origin is traced back to the prehistorical period when pigs, having been domesticated further to the east, were first introduced into Europe. It has lop ears.

Ukrainian Spotted Steppe

This small white black-spotted pig is an ancient breed which originated in the Ukraine. It has prick ears.

Vietnamese Pot Bellied

This relatively small pig, which tends to be obese as the name suggests, originated in Vietnam (Fig. 1.12). It also lives up to its name as it has a large pot belly. It can be black or mainly black with some white markings. It has a short snout and prick ears. It is the most popular pet pig in the UK.

Welsh

This small to medium-sized pig, as suggested by its name, originated in Wales. It is relatively rare now but is still bred in pedigree herds as it is often the basis of modern hybrid pigs.

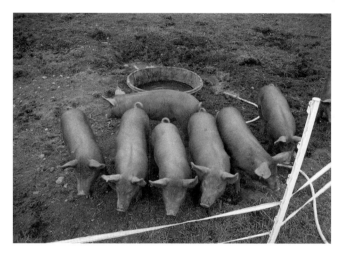

Fig. 1.11. Tamworth growing pigs.

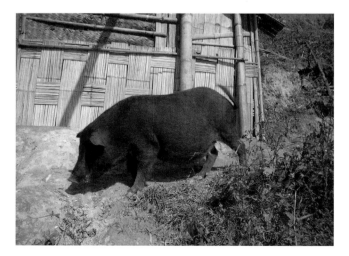

Fig. 1.12. A sow in north Vietnam.

West French White

This medium white pig is bred in France. It is an excellent bacon pig having a long back. It has lop ears.

Handling and Restraint

Baby pigs are easy to handle in a similar way to small dogs. They can be brought into the surgery in a cat basket (Fig. 1.13). It should be remembered that sows with suckling pigs can be extremely aggressive, therefore it is advisable to have the sow well contained and even out of earshot when handling her offspring (Fig. 1.14).

Commercial pig facilities normally have crates for handling sows and boars and weighing crates for handling fattening pigs. Some sort of crate is vital to contain adult pigs for handling and examination on smallholdings (Fig. 1.15). If a crate is not available, larger pigs can be controlled to some extent by pig boards. Weaner pigs can be controlled by holding their ears (Fig. 1.16). However, even very friendly pigs will endeavour to escape constantly. The ultimate method of control is a wire pig nose twitch or pig snare. This is placed on the upper jaw behind the canine teeth. The pig will try constantly to pull back and the wire, which is often in a hollow tube, should be kept under tension. Pet pig owners should be warned that pigs are very vocal but the noise is not in proportion to the pain. With big pigs owners should be warned of the danger of being bitten, savaged or knocked down.

Housing

Introduction

Housing for commercial pigs needs to be very sophisticated. For a smallholder in Laos, a bamboo stockade is fine (Fig. 1.17). Pet pigs in the UK can have very simple accommodation (Fig. 1.18). Accommodation costs are low for outdoor pigs (Fig. 1.19). However, outside pig arks need to be well maintained (Fig. 1.20). In Europe there is legislation limiting the tethering of pigs. Tethering pigs is a welfare issue (Fig. 1.21).

Space needs for growing pigs

This needs to be adjusted for the size of the pig. Normally the weight rather than the length is the parameter used. Values for outside pigs are shown in Table 1.1.

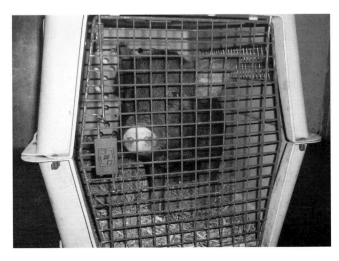

Fig. 1.13. Baby pigs can be brought into the surgery in a cat basket.

Health Planning

Herd health plans can be built around a checklist as shown in Table 1.2. A few of the differences between commercial, smallholder and pet pigs are highlighted. There are bound to be anomalies and each herd plan needs to be worked out on an individual basis between the pig owner and the practitioner. Small pig herds will have to decide whether they are to be considered as pets, small groups of pigs kept for home consumption (historically, backyard pig keepers kept four pigs from weaning to slaughter, three would be sold to pay for the food and the fourth would be eaten), breeding herds (catering for specialized meat production), pigs kept for rare breed survival or pigs kept for forest conservation. Pigs taken to agricultural shows are a

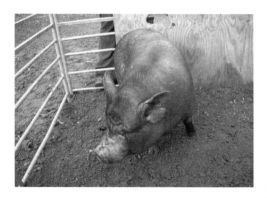

Fig. 1.14. A sow needs to be well contained.

potential zoonotic risk to the general public (Fig. 1.22). Also this practice should not be encouraged from a disease control point of view. The dangers of returning with a contagious disease are high. Pens of four pigs ready for slaughter are judged at Smithfield at Christmas. Obviously if these animals go on directly for slaughter, the home herd disease status is not compromised.

Health plans can be for the whole pig-keeping operation on a farm or they can be for specific areas, e.g. the farrowing accommodation, the weaner pool, etc. Or health plans can just be for a specific important disease, e.g. herd plans for *Salmonella*.

Waste Management

Manure in a commercial situation is relatively straightforward. If it is combined with straw it can be heaped and then spread on the land. Obviously this is easy if the arable land is being farmed in tandem with the pigs. If this is not the case, a linked deal of 'straw-for-muck' has to be arranged. If the pigs are outdoor pigs then their fields need to be rotated with arable fields in rotation. If pigs are on slats or have another slurry-type system, the slurry needs to be stored in a lagoon for later disposal. Whatever system is employed, manure needs to be removed on a really regular basis and stored well away from the pigs to prevent a problem with flies. With one or two pet pigs the manure can easily be mulched on

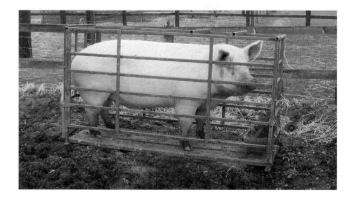

Fig. 1.15. Pigs need to have adequate restraint for examination.

to a muckheap and dug into a vegetable garden. Smallholders need to give thought to muck disposal.

Welfare Monitoring

Quality-oriented meat production has grown during the last decade and its aim is to improve the harmonization of product characteristics and consumer demands (Lambooij, 2012). Consumer concerns about quality are not limited solely to intrinsic characteristics, for example meat quality, but often include extrinsic aspects, such as environment and animal welfare in relation to production.

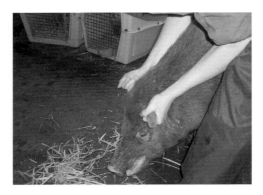

Fig. 1.16. Weaners can be controlled by holding their ears.

Post-mortem measurements in the slaughterhouse provide valuable information for welfare evaluation. The meat inspection process needs to be standardized. Lesions arising from tail biting could contribute to the surveillance of animal welfare on-farm (Harley *et al.*, 2012).

Pet Pigs

Introduction

The pig is becoming very popular as an outdoor and in some instances an indoor pet (Fig. 1.23). Pet pigs should be considered as companion animals. However, owners and veterinarians in the UK must remember that pet pigs require care like all farmed pigs and are subject to the various 'diseases of animals' legislation. Naturally they are also covered by any relevant 'welfare of animals' legislation. There are two traditional pet breeds, which are suitable for pet house-pigs. The most popular breed is the Vietnamese Pot Bellied Pig, sometimes called the Chinese House Pig. However, the Kunekune pig from New Zealand is growing in popularity. These breeds grow to approximately a quarter to half the size of a commercial pig. Given proper training they can make safe and friendly pets.

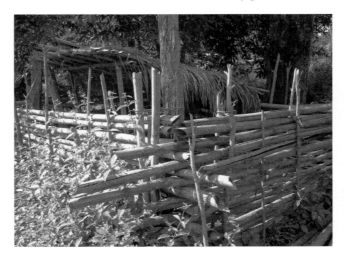

Fig. 1.17. A bamboo stockade.

Feeding and notifiable diseases

Feeding pet pigs is a major problem. First of all there is a potential very serious disease risk from feeding of household scraps. This should be strictly forbidden to avoid the risk of the spread of notifiable diseases, principally foot and mouth disease (FMD) and swine fever (SF). However, this rule is likely to be disobeyed by pet pig owners (Fig. 1.24). Therefore a pet pig might easily be the focus of an outbreak of FMD. It is necessary to clean

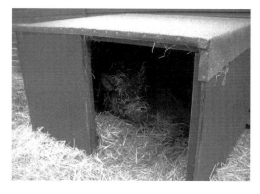

Fig. 1.18. Pet pig shelters can be simple.

the feet of pigs being examined to determine whether there are vesicular lesions present; it is important to use only clean water, as detergents and disinfectants will kill the FMD virus and make confirmation difficult. Vesicles are more common on the feet than on the tongue, lips or snout.

FMD should always be suspected if vesicular lesions are present, particularly if there is a high mortality in baby pigs. In older pigs morbidity is high but mortality is low.

The most common finding is the sudden onset of severe lameness. There is a high fever up to 41°C. The affected animals will have arched backs and be reluctant to move. If goaded they will squeal pitifully. They will be depressed and anorexic. The incubation period has been recorded as short as 2 days.

It must be remembered that a pig excretes 3000 times more virus particles than a cow, so it is vital that diagnosis is swift. Practitioners in the UK in any doubt should telephone the Department for Environment, Food and Rural Affairs (DEFRA) and stay on the holding until a Veterinary Officer (VO) arrives. If a practitioner is fairly sure that the problem is not FMD, but has just a slight doubt, then

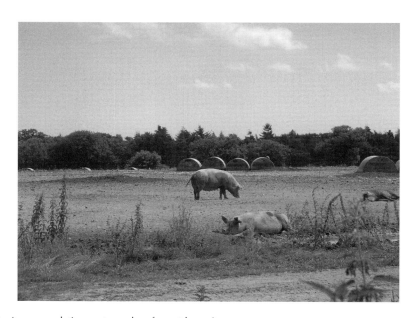

Fig. 1.19. Accommodation costs are low for outdoor pigs.

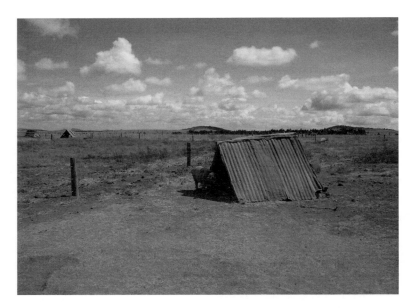

Fig. 1.20. Sharp tin is not acceptable even on a farm on the slopes of Mount Kenya.

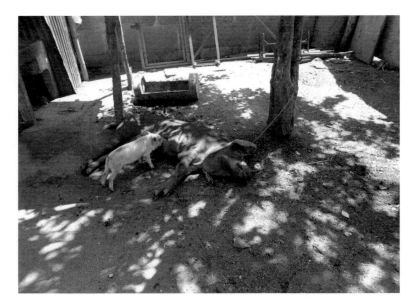

Fig. 1.21. This type of tethering is not acceptable.

there is no harm in telephoning another more experienced colleague in the practice or indeed from a neighbouring practice just to be on the safe side. However if FMD is suspected, obviously both practitioners must stay on the holding until a Government VO has arrived.

Exercise

Feeding is a problem for pet pig owners and obesity is extremely common. This is largely a problem in Pot Bellied pigs but can occur in Kunekune pigs. In the opinion of the author

Table 1.1. Space parameters for outside pigs.

	Weight of pig		
	Weaning to 35 kg	35–60 kg	>60 kg
Sleeping space or shelter per pig (m²)	1	1.5	2
Pigs per linear metre of self-feeder space	12	9	9
For hand feeding, running metre per pig	0.25	0.3	0.4

it is a major welfare issue. Pet pigs should be fed on proprietary prepared diets. Grazing and rooting should be encouraged. Exercise is important (Fig. 1.25). Rarely do owners walk their pigs. Naturally there is a disease risk to commercial pigs but paths can be found away from outside pigs. The code of practice issued by DEFRA is not strict but should be adhered to.

The owner may get permission to exercise a pet pig from the Divisional Veterinary Manager (DVM). The following rules will apply:

- An exact route must be specified and adhered to.
- The pig must be on a lead the whole time.
- There must be no contact with any other pig.
- The route must not go over agricultural land.
- The licence must be carried at the time of exercise.

Teeth

The pig at birth has 12 deciduous incisors, four deciduous canines (tusks) (Fig. 1.26) and 12 deciduous premolars. These are equally divided in the upper and lower jaws. They are all replaced by permanent teeth. They have 12 molars, which erupt later.

Reproduction

Pet pigs have the same reproductive parameters as commercial pigs. The length of gestation is 114 days with a normal variation of 2 days. The breeding cycles occur all year round, with oestrus occurring every 21 days with a variation of 1 day. Pet pigs normally have about six piglets in a litter (Fig. 1.27). It should be stressed to pet pig owners that breeding is a specialized affair and should not be carried out by amateurs. Castration should be advised at an early age unless the pigs are going for slaughter.

Environment

Real indoor pet pigs are rare. In these cases the minimum lying area should be 0.5 m² per 100 kg of pig, with an extra 1.5 m² for dunging and exercise. Most pet pigs are kept outside with a hut to provide some protection from the environment. A deep bed of straw is useful in winter and shade is essential in summer, a shallow water hole is beneficial (Figure 1.28).

Strong fencing is essential. Mains electric fencing is recommended to prevent the pigs rooting under a traditional fence. This rooting habit means that all electrical wires and water cables should be routed around the pig enclosure. Young pigs like to play with toys; they can be very destructive so toys and bowls etc. should be very robust. An area of concrete (not prepared with sharp gravel) is good to help the pig wear down the hooves naturally.

Manure disposal

Manure disposal is a difficult issue. On the one hand, the manure from one or two pigs can easily be mulched on a muckheap and dug into a vegetable garden. Equally, with a bigger operation the muck can be stored carefully and be taken away by a neighbouring farmer on a 'straw-for-muck' basis. It is the between-size operation where problems are likely to arise with not only the pig owner but

Table 1.2. Checklist for completion of a herd health plan.

Standard	Objective evidence
Traceability	The onus is on the pig keeper to record all movements either on or off the premises in the movement book. The pig keeper also has to record all medicines and their batch numbers given to the pigs
Tail docking	This is not advised and is permitted only on a written order from a veterinary surgeon that it needs to be performed on disease control grounds, for a limited period, until the situation is brought under control
Teeth clipping	This is no longer advised unless there is a specific problem. It should not be encouraged long term
Castration	This is not advised in a commercial situation. In a specific niche market where late maturing pig breeds are being kept, chemical castration should be considered (see Chapter 5, p. 48). Castration is advised only in pet pigs. In that situation the operation should be performed as early as possible at approximately 2 weeks of age
Prophylactic antibiotics	These are now banned in the EU and should be strongly discouraged in other areas of the world
Segregation of incoming pigs	This should be mandatory with as long an isolation period as possible
Welfare	A single person should be delegated as welfare officer. Any breaches of welfare standards should be recorded and new Standard Operating Procedures (SOPs) should be implemented as soon as possible
Regular inspection of pigs	Obligatory twice daily. More frequent inspections are required for parturient animals
Medicine record book	Obligatory
Knowledge of broken needle protocol	This should be available in writing (see below)
Withdrawal periods for medicines	These must be recorded for all medicines in the medicine record book. It should be remembered that any medicine used off licence has a meat withhold of 28 days
Records of births and deaths	This is strongly advised
Feed storage conditions	These should be checked weekly
Use of sticks, pipes or electric goads	Banned
Condition of structures and fittings	No sharp or broken gates or metal coverings
Condition of floors and bedding	Concrete to be checked monthly, bedding always to be adequate
Cleansing policy	A written good hygiene policy should always be followed
Temperature and ventilation	Adequate for each class of pig and able to be altered with extremes of weather conditions
Lighting	Adequate. Pigs must not live in darkness
Alarms	These are required only if there is mechanical temperature control practised. Smoke alarms are recommended
Pest control	Pigs must be kept vermin free. Bait must be protected from the pigs
Waste control	No excessive build-up of dung, particularly slurry
Water supply	This must be reliable even in severe frost
Piglet creep environment	This must be warm enough (see Housing section above)
Pig condition score	Pigs must not be too thin or obese. This is particularly relevant to pet pigs
Pig groups	Stability is important (practitioners should look for evidence of fighting)
Stocking density	Area must be sufficient for the number and size (see Housing section above)
Feeding space	Must be adequate (see Housing section above)
Level of antisocial behaviour and vice	Needs to be assessed with sympathy for the pigs and the pig keeper

Table 1.2. Continued.

Standard	Objective evidence
Treatment of sick pigs	Must be prompt with the ability to move into separate pens
Provision for euthanasia	This should be a written policy with veterinary involvement (see Chapter 6)
Drainage and land suitability	This is particularly important with outdoor pigs. The whole area occupied by the pigs should be checked visually
Standard and positioning of accommodation	This should be visually assessed
Electric fence training and acclimatization	This is relevant to outdoor pigs. Pig keepers should be educated
Wallows and shade	This is relevant to outdoor pigs and should be visually assessed
Nose ringing practice	This is no longer acceptable as it contravenes one of the five welfare freedoms
Weaning environment	This is one of the most stressful events in a pig's life. The environment should be visually appraised
Rotation of farrowing accommodation and location	Hygiene and education regarding straw burning

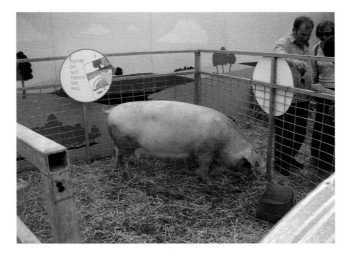

Fig. 1.22. Pigs at shows are a danger to the public.

also the neighbours. Careful commonsense education will have to be given.

Carcass disposal

Carcass disposal has to be regulated to fit in with current regulations and legislation. With small operations it would be suggested that disposal would be similar to domestic pets. However, with a larger operation and a larger number of pigs, a commercial carcass collector should be employed. His location and telephone number should be obtained before the need arises.

Legal requirements

Pet pigs are treated by DEFRA the same as commercial pigs. The owner is required to be registered with DEFRA and have a holding number.

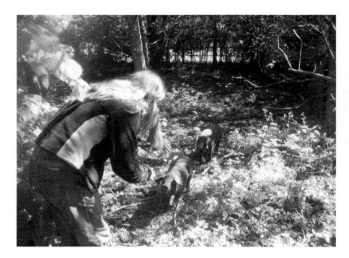

Fig. 1.23. Pigs make good outdoor pets.

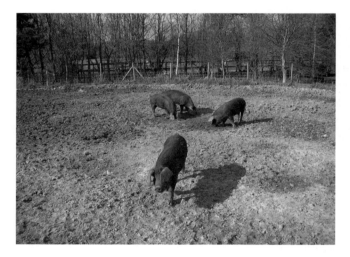

Fig. 1.24. Easy to throw scraps to these pigs kept at a children's care home.

The movement of all pigs must be recorded in an 'On Farm Movement Record'. This records the date the pigs were moved from or to the premises, the numbers moved, their identification marks and the address to or from which they have been moved. Welfare must be considered (Fig. 1.29).

No pigs should be moved off premises within 20 days of any pigs moving on to those premises. When pigs are moved off premises a movement licence must accompany them, which can be a signed declaration by the owner. When a self-issued declaration is issued, a copy should be sent to the local authority. Blank copies of declaration forms may be obtained from the Trading Standards department of the local authority or farming organizations such as the National Farmers' Union.

Pigs may be allowed to visit veterinary premises for emergency treatment, but the

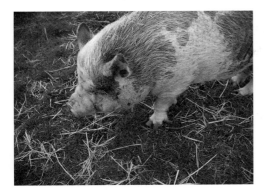

Fig. 1.25. Pigs benefit from walking on concrete to keep their hooves worn.

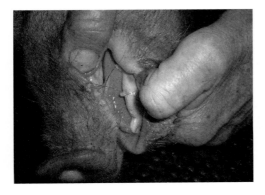

Fig. 1.26. A deciduous canine.

DVM needs to be informed as soon as possible if the regulations regarding pigs coming on to the holding within 20 days have not been adhered to. The vehicle needs to be thoroughly washed and disinfected with an approved disinfectant before and after the journey.

If pigs are carried in a vehicle loaded and unloaded just for the purpose of feeding and watering, there is no requirement to cleanse and disinfect the vehicle.

If pigs are moved under a movement declaration to a slaughterhouse, they must be slaughtered within 72 h. They cannot be removed alive from the slaughterhouse.

All persons in charge of premises receiving pigs must retain a copy of all movement declarations for 6 months.

It must be remembered that as pigs are a potential food-producing animal, a medicine book has to be kept by the owner. All medicines have to be recorded: the amount, name and batch number of the medicine, and the expiry date. The identification of the pig and the route of administration also have to be noted. Lastly, even though it may be abhorrent to the owner, the date when the pig is fit for human consumption has to be recorded.

A booklet giving advice on the legal aspects of owning pigs has been published by Animal Health. It is aimed at people who keep,

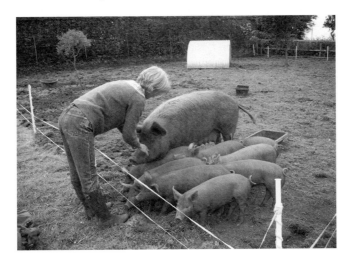

Fig. 1.27. A smallholder herd. A single sow and her litter.

or are considering keeping, pigs or 'micro' pigs as pets or as a hobby. This booklet can be downloaded from Animal Health's website (http://www.defra.gov.uk/ahvla-en/files/pub-pigs-micro-pet.pdf). This booklet gives advice on not only disease control but also animal welfare requirements. Points on feeding and biosecurity are also covered.

Handling

As stated earlier, baby pigs are easy to handle in a similar way to small dogs. It should be remembered that sows with suckling pigs

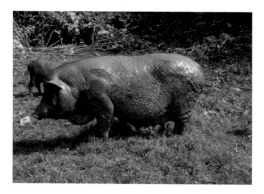

Fig. 1.28. Wallows are essential.

could be extremely aggressive; therefore it is advisable to have the sow well contained and maybe even out of earshot when handling her offspring.

Bigger pigs present a much harder handling problem. A strong person can lift a 35 kg pig by the hind legs; the ventral surface of the pig should be towards the handler. The handler's legs should grip the forequarters of the pig.

Although they are pets it is useful to have a crate of some type, e.g. a farrowing crate or an old weighing crate, to contain pigs for handling and examination. If a crate is not available then larger pigs can be to some extent controlled by pig boards. It should be remembered that even very friendly pigs will endeavour to escape constantly. The ultimate method of control is a wire pig nose twitch. This should be placed on the upper jaw behind the canine teeth. The pig will try constantly to pull back and the wire, which is often in a hollow tube, should be kept under tension. Owners should be warned that pigs are very vocal and the noise is not in proportion to the level of pain. With big pigs owners should be warned of the danger of being bitten, savaged or knocked down.

Examination of large pigs is not easy as they often resent handling. Quietness is vital for auscultation of the heart, lungs and abdomen. Patience will allow palpation of the abdomen,

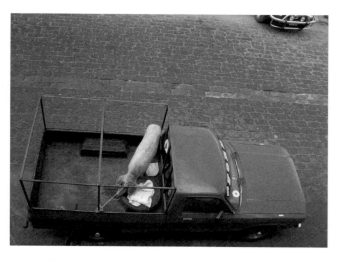

Fig. 1.29. Transport in Ecuador. This would be illegal in the UK.

mammary glands and feet. Rectal temperature is an extremely useful diagnostic sign in the pig; the normal is 39°C. The lack of hair allows a good examination of the pig's skin. Mucous membranes are best examined in the mouth, as the eyes are somewhat sunken. Pigs are highly intelligent animals; the owner's observations on behavioural changes and demeanour are well worth recording.

Abnormal Behaviour

Introduction

There are three main factors which contribute to abnormal behaviour in pigs. They are management, nutrition and disease. Management factors are the most common but least acceptable to pig keepers. Clinicians need considerable tact when dealing with these problems. Changes in management may be small and not expensive; equally they may be large and very costly. Clinicians need to be very sure of their diagnosis before advising on the latter course of action. Prudence would dictate that nutritional and disease problems are ruled out before costly changes are advised.

The effect of dietary inadequacy on pig welfare is seen particularly in early weaned pigs. Cheaper diets tend not to have ingredients which are palatable to newly weaned pigs. Reduced feed intake causes not only a slowing of growth rates but also increases behavioural problems.

Belly-nosing

Pigs have their rooting behaviour inhibited in fully slatted pens. It may also occur on solid floor pens which do not have any bedding. The provision of toys may be helpful in preventing the condition. The condition may predispose the pigs to contracting Greasy Pig Disease caused by *Staphylococcus hyicus*. Belly-nosing is more common in early weaned pigs, so sometimes even a delay of 48 h in weaning can reduce the behaviour.

Ear biting

This is more commonly seen in aggressive breeds. Removal of the sharp enamel points on the canine teeth soon after birth often does not help this vice, which is often seen soon after weaning. Poor palatability of diets tends to cause poor growth rate, unthriftiness and an increased attraction to blood. Low iron levels might also increase the attraction to blood. Nowadays all indoor pigs receive an injection of 1 ml of iron dextran soon after birth and so iron levels are adequate during the suckling period. However, if levels of iron in the creep are not adequate then pigs may show this vice in the immediate post-weaning period. Ear biting may be seen in pigs which have skin lesions as a result of porcine reproductive and respiratory syndrome (PRRS).

Penis sucking

This vice is nearly always seen soon after weaning. It may have a common aetiology to belly-nosing. It may lead to wet eczema of the sheath. Provision of solid floors, straw and toys are all thought to be helpful.

Urine drinking

This vice is commonly seen if there is inadequate provision of water. This may be because there are too few bowls or nipples or if there is insufficient pressure in the water supply to the nipples. The diagnosis needs to be made by careful observation. It is normally a vice of newly weaned pigs but can be seen in fattening pigs of any age.

Wall licking

There may be a possible link with several types of abnormal behaviour, often termed vices, to a diet low in salt. Ideally the diet should have 0.9% w/w NaCl. Provided there is an adequate supply of water, pigs can easily tolerate well above 1% w/w NaCl in their diet.

Animal Husbandry Procedures to Help Disease Control

'All-in, all-out'

Ideally this should apply to the whole farm. However, it may still be helpful by building, but is it is unlikely to be helpful just by pen. It must be strictly applied. There must be no half measures. 'All-in all-out' means just that.

Strict cleaning and disinfection procedures

These are vital in any system but particularly in an 'all-in all-out' system. Hygiene standards are absolutely critical. Pens should be wet down with detergent and left as long as possible to soak. ALL of the accessible organic material must be power-washed off. Then the whole pen must be disinfected with a suitable farm disinfectant used at the correct dilution as per instructions. The whole pen ideally should be dried first with a flame thrower and then with air movement. Microorganisms need water to survive, so drying is vital.

Limit the mixing of pigs

It is best to try to maintain pig groups from weaning right through to slaughter. Mixing pigs increases pig-to-pig contact and places pigs under stress. Both these factors increase the prevalence of disease.

Farrowing

Colostral immunity is very important. It is vital that piglets receive sufficient colostral uptake within the first 6 h. Colostrum intake should continue during the next 18 h. Cross-fostering should cease after 24 h as then there is a danger of a further spread of microorganisms. Ideally the immunity status of a group of piglets is fixed after 24 h. In many instances teeth clipping is unnecessary. It is vital to keep clippers as sterile as possible. Ideally several pairs should be on the go at any one time, so that the spare pairs can be stored in disinfectant. Needles for iron injections and any vaccinations should be regularly changed. One per litter should be considered as a minimum. Sows/gilts should be given a good wash and treated for parasites before entering the farrowing house. Parasitic burdens in the sow result in the animal becoming disadvantaged or in poor condition. In this state its colostrum levels might be compromised, having a detrimental effect on the piglets.

Partitions and pen size

All partitions between pens should be solid. Open partitions allow pig-to-pig contact, which allows the spread of disease. Nose-to-nose contact between pigs in different batches should be avoided at all costs. Lower stocking densities help reduce stress for the pigs, which in turn will increase health levels. Weaners should be no closer than three pigs per square metre, i.e. 0.6 m^2 per pig. Growers and finishers should be allowed 3.75 m per pig. Pen size groups should ideally be a whole litter, i.e. 13 pigs per pen. Pigs should have plenty of room to access feeders. Greater access lowers the need to fight for food and therefore lowers stress levels. Chilling also causes stress so temperatures should vary as little as possible.

Removal of pigs

Sick pigs should be removed promptly. The longer sick pigs are left in the pen, the greater the likelihood that other pigs in the pen will become sick. There should be a formalized sick-pig policy. It should be in writing and strictly adhered to. It should be clear when a pig should be euthanased or how long it will be given to recover. There is nothing more demoralizing than sick pigs not recovering. Guidelines should be clear, so that sick pigs will be destroyed before welfare is an issue. This will be good for staff morale. Dead pigs should be removed promptly to a remote area of the farm and then covered with straw pending disposal. The sight of dead pigs is very disturbing for staff and will not help morale. They act as a constant reminder of the problems.

Air quality

Air quality is important for welfare and to reduce the development of respiratory disease. NH_3 levels should be <10 ppm. CO_2 levels should be <0.15% w/w. Improving air flow within a building will help to reduce toxic gases. This will reduce stress on the respiratory system.

Broken Needle Policy

Introduction

Broken needles are rare, particularly if the correct length and gauge are used. The length required is not only dependent on the size of pig but also whether the injection has to go subcutaneously (sc), intramuscularly (im) or intravenously (iv). Obviously long needles are more likely to break than shorter needles. Breakage may occur mid-shaft or at the end near to the syringe. Breakage can occur in disposable syringes actually where the needle fits on to the syringe. When injecting adults or large pigs, pig keepers and practitioners are urged to use non-disposable syringes with a luer-lock fitting. The gauge of the needle will depend not only on the size of pig but also the viscosity of the fluid for injection. Long-acting preparations are notoriously viscous.

Length of needle

For adults and large pigs when injecting im a 4 cm needle is required. Weaners when injected im will require a 2.5 cm needle and piglets will require a 1 cm needle. For subcutaneous injection, e.g. when giving local anaesthetic above the mammary gland for a Caesarean section, a 5 cm needle will be useful so that it can be advanced slowly injecting local anaesthetic continuously up to its full length. This avoids repeated skin injections. For blood testing adults a 5 cm needle will be required for the jugular but a 2 cm needle will be more appropriate for an ear vein.

Gauge of needle

These are often colour coded. For a viscous liquid to be given im to an adult sow with some speed, a 14 gauge (orange) is useful. Often a 16 gauge (grey) is sufficient. For quiet sows or gilts an 18 gauge (pink) is adequate, particularly if the liquid is free flowing. For weaner pigs a 19 gauge (yellow) should be used. For piglets if the fluid is viscous a 21 gauge (green) is required, but if the liquid is free flowing a 23 gauge (blue) will be fine. For blood testing sows a 19 gauge (pink) should be used into the jugular but a 21 gauge (green) should be used in the ear vein. For blood testing gilts or weaners into the vena cava a 19 gauge (yellow) should be used. A 23 gauge (blue) will be adequate into the ear vein.

Needle breaks

If the metal piece is still visible:

- Restrain the pig immediately with a nose snare and remove the broken needle. Ideally a large pair of artery forceps should be kept sterilized ready for this eventuality. However a pair of pliers may be adequate.

If the metal piece is inside the pig and not visible:

- Immediately the pig should be marked with a numbered ear tag. The identity of the pig with the date should be recorded in the medicine book.

Possible future option for the animal if it is to be retained as breeding stock:

- The animal will not be suitable for human consumption.
- Ensure the animal tag is correctly placed.
- Check the animal's health regularly.

- Check the tag regularly and replace if necessary.
- If a different tag number is used, record the new number.
- Once the animal's breeding life is finished the animal must not go to slaughter for human consumption. The reason is that pieces of metal move inside the body and within a few weeks it will have moved from the injection site (i.e. the neck) to any part of the body. Practitioners should be very wary of trying to find the needle, even with ultrasound guidance, as it is extremely difficult and the welfare of the pig will be compromised.

If the pig is of adequate size and has not received medicine which has too long a meat withhold, it can be slaughtered within 7 days:

- The animal should be sent to a slaughterhouse.
- It should be accompanied by an owner's declaration for casualty slaughter.
- The slaughterhouse should be advised as to the injection site.

The pig may be finished for home consumption:

- The pig once finished MUST NOT BE SOLD.

If the pig cannot be slaughtered within 7 days, has no breeding future and cannot be used for home consumption:

- The pig should be destroyed humanely.

All needles, syringes and containers should be disposed of according to legal requirements.

Herd Recording

Introduction

Recording and measuring the performance of pig herds, particularly breeding herds, is vital to gauge herd performance and subsequent profitability. Key indicators include: number born alive, piglet survival and kilograms of meat sold per sow per year. These need to be compared with the national average and hopefully with the top 10% of the national pig herds.

More specific indicators, which should be linked to targets, need to be recorded in breeding herds.

Farrowing rate

The farrowing rate tells you the number of sows that farrow as a percentage of the number of sows and gilts that are served. The target should be 85% (more in an elite herd). This means that for every 100 sows and gilts which are served, 85 have gone on to farrow, while the remaining 15 have returned to service, been culled or died. It is vital that there is a record kept of all farrowings over a 12-month period. This figure is then divided by the total number of sows and gilts served. The answer is then multiplied by 100. The farrowing rate can be tracked monthly by deleting data from the earliest month and adding data from the latest month. For a real-time farrowing rate record, draw up a fertility chart and record weekly services, subsequent failures and expected farrowing rate percentage. This will allow a quicker response if things start to go wrong.

Obviously any new disease problems will lower the farrowing rate. However, there are other factors which will affect the farrowing rate and will need to be addressed in a diplomatic manner with the management and the pig keepers:

- Sow and gilt management (stable body conditions and social environments are particularly important).
- Nutrition and feeding regimens.
- Stockmanship (heat observation, heat recording, service/artificial insemination (AI) management and handling techniques are very important).
- Physical environment (thermal environment and hygiene are very important).
- Culling decisions.

The farrowing rate gives a guide to how many sows you need to serve to run the farrowing accommodation at optimum capacity. This is important not only from the viewpoint of physical use of the farrowing house or the farrowing arks, but also maximizing the output from the labour force. As an example, if the farrowing accommodation is sufficient for 160 sows and there is a farrowing rate of 85%, then there will be a need to serve 190 sows each week.

Farrowing index

The farrowing index is literally the number of litters per sow per year. The target should be 2.25. This can be raised to 2.4 in really elite herds. The farrowing index is determined by four key factors:

- The length of pregnancy (this could be as short as 114 days but might creep up to 117 days).
- The length of lactation (this is problematic in the UK as the legal age for weaning of piglets is 28 days).
- The length of time it takes for normal sows to return to oestrus after weaning (this is normally 6 days but may be shorter particularly with the correct use of hormone injection; see Chapter 10).
- The so-called non-productive days.

Non-productive days

Realistically, the main target to improve the farrowing index is to reduce the number of non-productive days. The factors to concentrate on are:

- To avoid any delay after weaning for the sow returning to oestrus (e.g. thin sows or poor boar exposure).
- To avoid missing a service. Services may be missed if the sow actually comes on heat in the farrowing accommodation or if there is poor oestrus detection.

- To avoid sows returning to service at the normal/expected time. This is easy to say but very hard to prevent. Obviously there may be a pathogen involved (see Chapter 10), which will need addressing after a diagnosis, but this is unlikely if the return is at the expected time. There may be a poor service environment. Timing of service is important whether this is natural service or AI.
- To avoid sows having a return to service at a longer time than expected. This is most likely to be caused by a pathogen. A diagnosis and a treatment plan is then a priority.
- To avoid culling or dying. This is a crass statement but actually with careful planning this is possible with various disease control strategies, e.g. reducing lameness by attention to the flooring, reducing deaths by vaccination. It is therefore very important that the reason for culling is recorded and obviously with any deaths the reason is recorded.

Pre-weaning mortality

This should be less than 10% and mortality due to scour in sucking pigs, less than 0.5%. Different diseases typically affect piglets at different ages; hence it is important to record the ages at which pigs are noted to be scouring, are treated and die. Many of the causes of scour in sucking piglets will damage or destroy the all-important villi in the small intestine, which are responsible for absorption of nutrients. Loss of these villi will predispose piglets to post-weaning scours because nutrients which should be absorbed in the small intestine can end up feeding the bacteria present in the large intestine, leading to bacterial proliferation there and scour.

2 Nutrition

Introduction

Pigs are omnivores. Wild species in their natural environment eat a very wide variety of foodstuffs. Domesticated pigs are kept in very varied environments from extremely large commercial breeding and fattening units through to smallholder units with pigs living very closely with humans in rural environments, to pet pigs living very close to their owners. Their nutrition will vary in a similar manner, with very high scientific diets and at the lower range ad hoc diets. In all situations it should be stressed that pigs should NEVER be fed any household scraps containing meat products because of the danger of the spread of pandemic infectious diseases, e.g. FMD, classical swine fever (CSF) and African swine fever (ASF). In most countries these diseases are notifiable and there is legislation banning not only the feeding of household scraps but also the feeding of commercial waste products called swill.

The full nutritional requirements for all types, ages and breeds of pig are beyond the scope of this book. Diseases of the neurological system and the skin as they are related to nutrition are listed below and also will be cross-referenced in Chapters 11 and 12.

Water

Good-quality water must be freely available even if pigs are being fed wet feed. This includes suckling pigs. These require 60 ml/kg daily. Weaners weighing 15 kg require 2 l daily. Fat pigs weighing 90 kg require 12 l daily. Non-pregnant sows require 12 l daily, pregnant sows require 20 l daily and lactating sows require 40 l daily. This is an important welfare requirement. Interruption of water availability will cause the acute neurological problem of salt poisoning.

Food Requirements

Nutritional deficiencies and excesses

These are rarely a problem in well-run commercial herds. They only become a problem when errors occur, e.g. in mixing of food when home mixing is carried out or spillage of food when moulds may become a problem; lack of cleaning of food bins will also add to this problem. When pigs escape there are likely to be problems with excess food and toxicity from eating garbage, etc. Nutritional problems are much more common in smallholder operations, e.g. when too much bread is fed from bakery waste. Practitioners should question pig keepers carefully in a no-blame manner to see if nutritional requirements of pigs have been met. Any bought food should be examined carefully for any physical problems. If need be, samples may be taken for analysis.

In the commercial world the genetics of pigs are constantly being upgraded. It is important that diets are constantly reviewed as well.

Minerals

The total requirements are regularly revised. The minerals normally listed are: calcium, cobalt, copper, iodine, iron, magnesium, manganese, phosphorus, potassium, selenium, sodium and zinc.

Vitamins

As with minerals, the levels required are constantly being reviewed. The normal vitamins quoted are: vitamin A, vitamin D_3, vitamin E, vitamin C, vitamin K, vitamin B_{12}, thiamin, riboflavin, nicotinic acid, pantothenic acid, pyridoxine, choline, biotin and folic acid.

Amino acids

The requirement of essential amino acids is an emerging science. The two which are normally quoted are linolenic acid and arachidonic acid. However, new information is constantly being made available.

Pigs in the late finisher stage are often growing quickly towards market weight, at approximately 1 kg/day, with much of this growth being muscle development. This necessitates high levels of amino acid (AA) intake and uptake, and requires dietary attention to both high-protein feed components (such as soybean or fish meal) and also an AA feed supplement, particularly the first-limiting AAs lysine and threonine. Many commercial synthetic AA supplements contain lysine, threonine and other components. Incorporation of some larger muscled pig breeds, such as the

Pietrain, into farm breeding programmes may lead to higher incremental needs for these supplements. The usage of the metabolic partitioning agent ractopamine in some markets (non-European) plays a further major incremental role in this AA uptake requirement (Corona *et al.*, 2012).

Finisher feed costs are widely recognized as the major factor in the cost of the production of market pigs. The rapidly rising costs and diminishing availability of some of the high-protein components of these feeds have led to a search for strategies to reduce the necessity for excessive lysine and other AA intakes (Niven *et al.*, 2006). The numerous enterobacteria, such as those located in the pig intestine, can act to decarboxylate AA, producing biogenic amines such as cadaverine (Santos, 1998; Marino *et al.*, 2000). One of these lysine-conserving strategies is, therefore, to identify feed additives that may reduce the bacterial degradation of AA intake during their passage in the gastrointestinal (GI) tract. The sanguinarine alkaloids (derived from *Macleaya cordata* and related plants) were developed in the 1980s and 1990s for incorporation into a variety of commercial oral anti-inflammatory products. More recent development of these alkaloids has been for animal feed additives, partly as an anti-inflammatory agent (Chaturvedi *et al.*, 1997). Also, an *in vitro* study suggested an ability of these alkaloids to reduce the activity level of AA degradation enzymes, such as decarboxylase, located within the GI tract (Drsata *et al.*, 1996). However, investigation of the activity of these alkaloids within feed additives, aimed at reducing the degradation of dietary tryptophan during its passage through the pig, found no useful influence on performance (Blank *et al.*, 2010). Further research needs to be carried out to make certain these substances are really worthwhile in pig diets.

Nutritional induced diarrhoea

Naturally, clinicians should make sure that the diarrhoea has no infectious cause. Probably the most common non-infectious cause of diarrhoea is an imbalance of cereals, particularly a high wheat inclusion. Also new crop cereals, particularly barley, may cause problems. The reason for these problems is the presence of non-starch polysaccharides. These are xyloses and arabinoses, which are not digestible by pigs unless cooked. In the raw state they pass through the small intestine and absorb water. When they reach the large intestine they are altered by bacteria and release the water. The pig is not able to absorb all this and so diarrhoea occurs. The excessive use of soy meal to increase protein levels may cause colitis. Pig keepers are always complaining about high levels of manioc. However, there is little real evidence that manioc does cause colitis. There is evidence that rape meal in excess will cause colitis. The proven level is over 5% w/w of the diet. Such a high level is extremely unlikely unless there is a real mistake at the feed mill. Of course, an excessive feed intake will cause diarrhoea.

Colostrum

The importance of colostrum to the neonatal pig cannot be overstated. Adequacy of colostrum quantity and quality can and should be measured by blood testing piglets. The test used is the zinc turbidity test. Gilt colostrum is liable to be of poorer quality than that of sows,

so it is important to evaluate gilt colostrum by blood testing pigs from gilts as well as from sows. Milk continues to play an important role in providing antibodies to the mucus layer of the gut, which protects against infection. It is important that lactating gilts and sows are given adequate nutrition as well as access to fresh clean water at all times. Piglets reared away from a sow will survive if given adequate colostrum (Fig. 2.1).

Neurological Diseases Caused by Changes in Nutrition

Copper deficiency myelopathy

This is extremely rare. It may be associated with iron deficiency in commercial indoor pigs. Pigs may be found dead or convulsing from heart damage.

Copper toxicity

This is now rare as copper is no longer used as a growth promoter. Signs are anorexia and depression. The signs disappear rapidly when excess copper is removed from the diet.

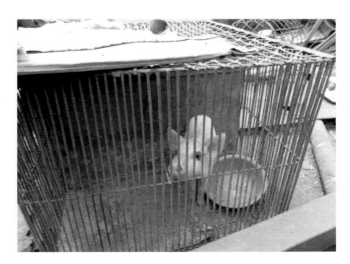

Fig. 2.1. Piglets reared away from a sow will survive if given adequate colostrum.

Hypoglycaemia

This is seen in neonatal pigs which have not received adequate energy, e.g. in very cold conditions when a sow has farrowed outside in winter. Convulsions will be seen in piglets. Hypoglycaemia can also be brought on by low levels of various infections in piglets. The farrowing fever complex syndrome, which will decrease milk output, will put piglets at risk. Treatment is proprietary energy fluids by mouth or in extreme cases injections of 15 ml of 5% w/w glucose intraperitoneally (ip) every 4 h.

Osteomalacia

This condition will mainly be seen in very badly fed adult, aged backyard pigs. Calcium has to be virtually absent from the diet. The bones are very brittle. The pig may have multiple long-bone fractures and be unable to rise (Fig. 2.2). Prompt euthanasia is the only course of action.

Vitamin A deficiency

This will cause blindness and so the pigs will appear to show nervous signs. The condition is certainly a possibility in badly fed backyard pigs. Once there is blindness recovery is impossible, even with vitamin A injections. Single or pairs of affected pigs might be thought to have a reasonable quality of life but euthanasia should be seriously considered.

Vitamin B deficiency

This may occur in backyard pigs fed either a very fatty diet or solely on bread. Normally pigs go off their hind legs; this is followed by a progressive paralysis. They may recover with good nursing and a proper diet.

Vitamin K deficiency

This occurs as a result of eating rat bait containing warfarin.

Skin Diseases Caused by Changes in Nutrition

Biotin deficiency

The main signs are hair loss and hoof lesions. Normally hoof lesions precede hair loss. Treatment with biotin in the food readily controls the condition and can be used as a diagnostic tool.

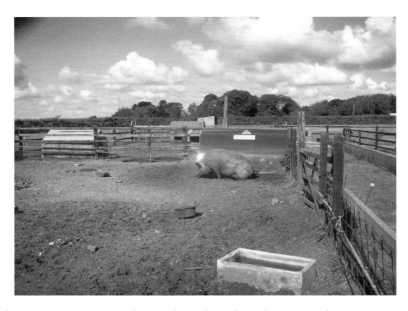

Fig. 2.2. This pig is not receiving an adequate diet and is suffering from osteomalacia.

Iodine deficiency

This is an extremely rare condition of piglets born to iodine-deficient sows. The piglets will be hairless but will not show goitre.

Parakeratosis

This is caused by a deficiency of zinc in the diet or by a conditioned deficiency from high levels of phytic acid in soy. It is found in young growing pigs and is manifest as scaly papules. Diagnosis should be made with a skin biopsy as testing the blood for zinc levels is unreliable. Treatment is restoring the zinc level in the diet to 100 ppm taking into account the level of soy in the food. The response to treatment can be used as a diagnostic tool.

Vitamin A deficiency

This is extremely rare and is manifest as a generalized seborrhoea. It is seen in weak piglets born to deficient sows. Other signs of vitamin A deficiency, e.g. neurological signs, particularly blindness, are going to be much more obvious than the skin disease. The neurological signs are irreversible.

Vitamin B deficiency

Other than biotin deficiency, which is relatively common, deficiencies of niacin, pantothenic acid and riboflavin have been reported as well but they are extremely rare. Skin disease signs are very variable but are usually seen as dry scaly areas. Total recovery will occur if the diet is corrected.

3 Making a Diagnosis and Post-mortem Technique

Clinical Examination

Examination of large pigs is not easy as they resent handling. Pigs need to be kept out of arks to examine them (Fig. 3.1). Quietness is vital for auscultation of the heart, lungs and abdomen. This is difficult to attain in most situations. Patience will allow palpation of the abdomen, mammary glands, limbs and feet. Rectal temperature is extremely useful in the pig. Reference levels for the clinical examination are given in Table 3.1.

The lack of hair allows a good examination of the skin, particularly in white pigs. This is obviously helpful for actual skin disease. It is also helpful with the diagnosis of many systemic diseases either because these diseases have specific signs on the skin, e.g. erysipelas, or because there are changes of colour of the skin, e.g. cyanosis in PRRS ('blue ear disease').

Diagnostic Laboratory Tests

Blood sampling

Obtaining blood samples is not easy from any age of pig. Piglets weighing <10 kg are best held in dorsal recumbency on the lap of a sitting person, who holds the front legs firmly with the head towards the veterinary surgeon.

The surgeon then holds the piglet's head in one hand and directs the 25 mm needle from the jugular groove in a caudo-medial direction into the anterior vena cava.

Older pigs are also best bled from the anterior vena cava with the nose held up in a pig snare. The blood vessel cannot be seen or palpated but the needle has to be directed medially from the indentation at the base of the neck.

Only in adults can blood be drawn from the jugular vein. The animal is best restrained in a crate with the head held as high as possible by the snare. The needle must be at least 38 mm long and should be directed at 45° in a dorso-medial direction from the caudal end of the jugular furrow. Blood can be drawn in adults with large ears from an ear vein. A tourniquet of a thick rubber band and a pair of artery forceps is placed at the base of the ear. The small veins can be seen on the outside of the ear between the skin and the cartilage. Blood can be drawn using a 23 mm needle on the end of a syringe to apply a small amount of suction.

Normal haematological and biochemical parameters are given in Tables 3.2 and 3.3.

Saliva

Saliva is an interesting tool because of its potential to reflect both oral and systemic

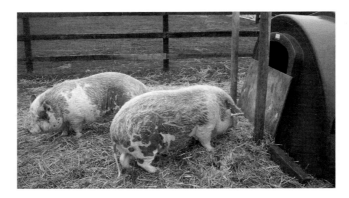

Fig. 3.1. The pigs need to be kept out of their house to examine them.

Table 3.1. Reference levels for the clinical examination of pigs.

Parameter	Values
Body temperature	Lower critical point, 38.4°C; normal, 39°C; upper critical point, 40°C
Pulse	70–80 beats/min, rising to 250 beats/min in the newborn piglet
Respiration rate	Adults, 10–20 breaths/min; growers, 20–30 breaths/min; newborns, 40–50 breaths/min

Table 3.2. Normal haematological parameters in pigs.

Parameter	Normal range
Packed cell volume (PCV)	37–46%
Red blood cells (RBCs)	6.5–8.0×10^{12}/l
White blood cells (WBCs)	10.0–23.0×10^9/l
Platelets	250–700×10^9/l
Haemoglobin (Hb)	11.0–14.2 g/dl

health conditions and, with the advent of proteomics, biomarkers can be identified for specific pathological disease processes to help in the early detection of disease in farm animals. A study in Spain (Guiterrez *et al.*, 2012) discovered potential salivary markers for systemic disease in pigs. Saliva samples can be obtained by allowing the pig to chew on a sponge for 2 min. Serological results can show positive results for PRRS, swine influenza virus (SIV) and porcine circovirus type 2 (PCV-2).

Urine samples

Obtaining urine samples requires considerable patience by the pig keeper. If required by the practitioner, catheterization of sows restrained in a crate is not difficult with a canine oesophageal tube. It is impossible to catheterize male pigs and so practitioners have to rely on a free-flowing sample. Normal urine parameters are as follows:

- Specific gravity (SG), 1.020.
- pH, 5.5–7.5.
- Protein and sugar, none.

Bacteriological examination of the urine can also be useful. Care needs to be exercised as certain bacteria will be grown as contaminates. The clinician will have to evaluate the bacteriological findings in the light of the clinical signs to decide from where in the urinary tract the bacteria originate.

Diagnostic Imaging

Radiography

Ten years ago radiography would not have featured in a book on pig surgery. That is not the case today, when we regularly radiograph pigs' legs. Good restraint and normally a general anaesthetic (GA) are required (Fig. 3.2). Radiographs are useful for: fractures, arthritic joints, sand cracks and septic joints. Obviously this is not in a commercial situation, but radiographs are very useful to aid not only in making a diagnosis but also in making a prognosis. The author finds the procedure extremely useful when dealing with rescued pigs in sanctuaries so that unnecessary suffering is avoided.

Head radiographs are useful for diagnosis of cheek teeth disorders. The author expects radiographs in pigs to be used more frequently in the future, particularly for pet pigs.

Ultrasonography

As yet ultrasonography has had limited use in pigs. With the advent of much loved pet pigs this may change. At the present time its

Table 3.3. Normal biochemical parameters in pigs.

Parameter	Mean	Range	Units
Calcium	2.70	2.4–3.0	mmol/l
Phosphorus	2.68	2.1–3.0	mmol/l
Sodium	152	133–171	mmol/l
Potassium	5.49	4.5–6.5	mmol/l
Chloride	No data available	95–110	mmol/l
Bilirubin	2.1	0.1–4.1	mmol/l
Total protein	70.4	55.84–85.4	g/l
Urea	5.5	2.9–8.1	mmol/l
Glucose	5.18	4.0–6.36	mmol/l
Lactate	5.2	0–11.0	mmol/l
Alkaline phosphatise (ALP)	215	140–290	IU/l
Aspartate aminotransferase (AST)	17	9–25	IU/l
Creatine kinase (CK)	No data available	0–800	IU/l
Cholesterol	No data available	2.0–3.3	mmol/l
γ-Glutamyl transferase (GGT)	No data available	10–40	IU/l
Glutamate dehydrogenase (GLDH)	No data available	0–5.5	IU/l

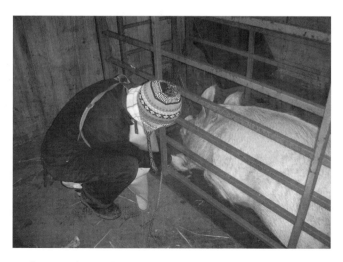

Fig. 3.2. Adult sow under general anaesthetic restrained for radiography.

use is restricted to pregnancy diagnosis and for visualization of stones lodged in the small intestine.

Post-mortem Examination

Equipment required

These articles are not normally carried by an ambulatory clinician:

- Large plastic bucket with disinfectant, warm water, soap and towel.
- Butcher's knife and flaying knife.
- Scalpel and blades that fit.
- Rat-toothed forceps (15 cm).
- Fine forceps (15 cm).
- Blunt-nosed straight scissors (20 cm).
- Bowel scissors.
- Bone cutters, saw and hedge loppers.

Post-mortem sampling materials required:

- Plastic trays (50 cm × 30 cm × 5 cm).
- Plastic bags of various sizes.
- Sterile universal bottles.
- Plastic jars (1 l).
- Bottles of formalin (kept separate).
- Pots containing 50% w/w glycerol for virus isolation.
- Swabs (plain, transport media and specialized media for respiratory pathogens).
- Pasteur pipettes and rubber suckers.
- Clipboard.
- Post-mortem report form, laboratory submission form.

Specific history required for post-mortem carcasses

The clinician needs to know if the pig was found dead or whether euthanasia was performed. It is useful to know how euthanasia was performed as shooting will damage the central nervous system (CNS) and lethal injections, if given into the heart, will damage the thorax. The length of time since death should be ascertained and how the body was managed in that time, i.e. fresh, chilled or frozen. The age, breed and weight should be recorded.

Before post-mortem the outside of the pig should be examined

The general appearance and colour should be noted. Careful examination should be made for the presence of ectoparasites, mainly lice and crusts relating to mange. Lice will often leave a dead pig, so their absence does not mean they were not present in life. Any crusts should be retained and can be supplemented with deep skin scrapings and even punch biopsies to help get a diagnosis.

At the start the head should be examined; is the snout twisted? Is there ocular discharge? Then the body; are there udder swellings? Is the prepuce normal? Are the feet and coronary band normal? Is the rectum/vulva normal?

Single-handed post-mortem technique without a cradle

This is easiest if carried out in a series of steps.

1. Lie the pig on its left side and make a bold cut in the axilla, cutting all the skin and musculature so that the right front leg is totally reflected on to the ground.
2. Make a bold cut into the groin into the adductor muscles going straight into the hip joint and severing the ligament anchoring the femoral head into the acetabulum, so that right hind leg can be totally reflected (Fig. 3.3). The carcass should now be stable on its side.
3. Cut the skin from the opening around the hind leg along the ventral mid-line to the skin cut in the axilla (Fig. 3.4).
4. Cut the skin from this skin incision through the ventral mid-line, reflect the skin as a large flap to the spine so that it can be laid out behind the backbone as a flat surface with the skin on the ground. This can then be used to lay the internal organs on, rather than on the ground.
5. Cut the skin from the cranial point of the ventral skin incision, an incision should be made cranially to the symphysis of the mandibular rami.
6. Cut the skin from the caudal point of the ventral skin incision, an incision should be made caudally to the rectum/vulva.

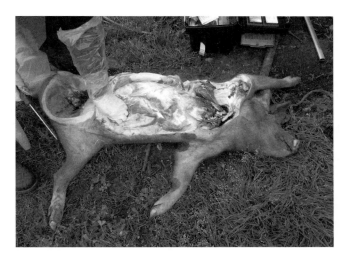

Fig. 3.3. The upper and lower legs are reflected.

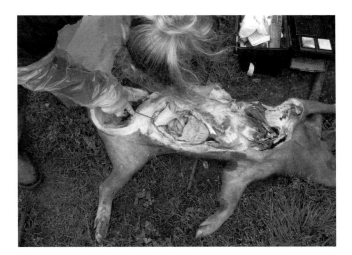

Fig. 3.4. The abdomen is opened.

7. The abdominal cavity should be opened carefully from the xiphisternum to the pubic symphysis. Samples can be taken from the peritoneal fluid and from the liver for bacteriology.

8. The abdominal musculature should be cut along the line of the last rib from the xiphisternum to the spine, so that the flank can be reflected and the internal organs revealed (Fig. 3.5). The liver will just be seen caudal to the xiphisternum with a small portion of the stomach. The rest of the abdomen will be filled with the greater omentum cranially and the jejunum caudally.

9. Two cuts should now be made through the diaphragm along both costalchondral junctions cranially and including the first ribs. In growing and fattening pigs these cuts can normally be carried out with a sharp post-mortem knife. In adults a saw or a pair of garden loppers may be required. Then the whole sternum can be removed.

10. Multiple cuts should be made through the intercostal muscles between the ribs dorsally to the spine, so that each rib can be broken in a dorsal direction near to the spine. The heart, lungs and the rest of the thorax can

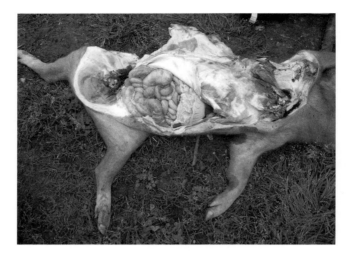

Fig. 3.5. The liver, spleen, small and large bowel are visible.

then be examined *in situ*. Bacteriological samples can be taken at this stage. Heart blood can be aspirated.

11. A cut should be made between the mandibles so that the tongue can be grasped. It should be pulled using blunt dissection so that the whole 'pluck' can then be removed, i.e. the larynx, trachea, oesophagus, lungs and heart.

12. A cut at the caudal end of the oesophagus will remove the 'pluck' from the intestinal tract.

13. A cut should be made down both the trachea and the oesophagus to examine the internal mucosa.

14. The lungs, the mediastinal lymph nodes and the thymus should be examined carefully. The pericardium, the outside and the inside of the heart should be examined, paying particular attention to the heart valves.

15. The whole intestinal tract should be examined outside and inside. This should also include an examination of the liver, spleen, omentum and lymph nodes. The contents of the intestinal tract should be examined for nematodes and samples should be taken for bacteriology.

16. The rest of the carcass should be examined. This should include the adrenal glands, kidneys, ureters, bladder and urethra. Bacteriological samples can be taken at this stage. The uterus or male genital tract should also be examined. The contents of the bladder

should be examined and a sterile sample should be taken if required.

Two-person post-mortem technique or single-handed technique using a cradle

The pig is laid in dorsal recumbency with the helper holding one leg to keep it upright or laid in the cradle. A skin incision is made from the chin straight down the ventral surface all the way to the anus. A small incision is carefully made through the abdominal musculature and the peritoneum caudal to the xiphisternum. This incision is then lengthened caudally to the pubic symphysis, making sure that the internal organs are not cut. Two cuts are made from the xiphisternum cranially through the costalchondral junctions so that the sternum can be removed. The internal organs can then be examined *in situ*. Bacteriological samples can be taken at this stage. The pluck and the intestinal tract can then be removed as described above.

The internal organs etc. to be examined in the abdominal cavity are: the umbilicus together with the whole internal peritoneal surface, the liver including the gall bladder, the spleen, kidneys and adrenals, the ureters, bladder and urethra, the uterus, fallopian tubes, ovaries and mammary glands, the testes, vesicular gland, bulbourethral glands and the penis.

The alimentary tract can be examined starting with: the tongue, lips, teeth, pharynx and oesophagus, the stomach (noting contents), the duodenum, jejunum and ileum, the colon, caecum and rectum, the mesenteric lymph nodes and the pancreas.

The respiratory tract and thoracic cavity can be examined starting with: the snout and turbinates, the larynx, trachea and lungs, the heart, thymus and mediastinal lymph nodes.

The neurological system can be examined after the cranium and the spinal column have been opened. Bacteriological samples can be taken at this stage. The brain, spinal column and peripheral nerves should all be examined.

Carcass disposal

Carcasses from post-mortem examinations (PMEs) must be disposed of safely and hygienically. Post-mortems should be performed on washable surfaces so that surface water and ditches are not contaminated. The post-mortem shown in Figs 3.3 to 3.5 is far from ideal. Carcasses need to be buried in a deep covered pit at least 4 m from a watercourse (these are no longer allowed in the UK) or incinerated. If carcasses are to be picked up by a knacker-man or an agent of the Fallen Stock Scheme (this only operates in the UK), they should be dragged to a specially prepared concrete area on the outside of the holding so there is no need for a possibly contaminated vehicle to enter the holding. Ideally this should be a building which can then be refrigerated. It should have appropriate drainage and be capable of cleansing and disinfection.

4 Veterinary Equipment

Equipment for Handling

Naturally a bucket, brush, farmyard disinfectant, rubber boots and waterproofs are required.

You must not only be clean but also look clean. If there is a spray for cleaning your car wheels, use it. If there are foot dips on the farm, use them. If the farm provides clean boots and overalls, use them. If it provides plastic disposable over-boots, use them.

A strong rope, 5 m in length, is required for securing adult pigs to a fixed gate. Some 2 m × 2 m lengths of thin rope are required to help with restraint of an adult pig's legs when it is in a crate. A pig snare is a vital requirement (Fig. 4.1).

Equipment for Diagnosis

Arm-length sleeves are required for internal examinations but are probably not used for actual parturition procedures. A digital camera is important so that the clinician has the ability to take pictures and download the photographs, label them, store them, and send them as attachments to e-mails. A stethoscope is required but it is not as useful as in other species. Various types of swab are required. Some should have transport media and some plain. A clinical thermometer is vital.

The traditional glass thermometers will last for years if kept carefully in a plastic case. They are hard to acquire in the UK because of the mercury content. However, there are digital thermometers available. The clinician needs to choose whether the thermometer reads Centigrade or Fahrenheit. It is just a matter of which the clinician is happy with.

In pet pig practice often pigs are either seen in the hours of darkness or are contained in a dark hut. A head torch is useful on these occasions. It is also useful for dentistry (see below).

Equipment for Treatment

A variety of hypodermic needles of different sizes with luer fitting are required. A variety of disposable syringes of different sizes are needed with luer mounts. Practitioners also require a strong, non-disposable plastic syringe with a luer-lock needle fitting. A large, all-metal needle is required to avoid the risk of a broken needle. This is for injecting unrestrained pigs (Fig. 4.2).

There are automatic injection systems which allow up to 20 ml to be injected im from up to 1.5 m away. These are very effective. Some practitioners inject unrestrained pigs by the use of a piece of extension tubing connected between the needle and the syringe.

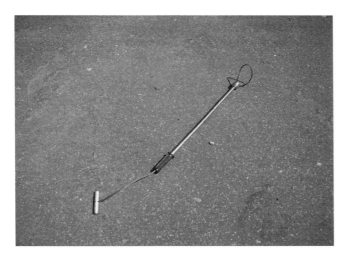

Fig. 4.1. A pig snare.

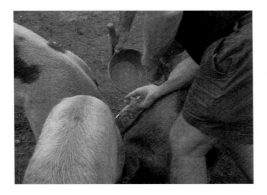

Fig. 4.2. Non-disposable syringe for a rapid injection.

The pig is jabbed and then the drug is injected by the practitioner following behind. The advantage is that if the pig breaks away, the needle can be pulled out and not left *in situ*. The author has had only variable success with this procedure as often the needle is dislodged too early.

Spinal needles 15 cm in length with luer fitting are required for euthanasia. A 25 cm seaton needle with uterine tape is needed to place a 'Buhner suture' for vaginal and uterine prolapses. A 15 cm curved cutting edged suturing needle with braided nylon suture material is required for purse string sutures in pigs with rectal prolapses.

Equipment for the Feet

Hoof knife

The type of knife is a very individual choice. Obviously there are knives for left and right hands. Equally there are double-sided knives which can be used in either hand. The looped knives are useful for removing the softer parts of the hoof.

Hoof trimmers

The large size is required for adult pigs (Fig. 4.3).

Gutter tape

A roll of this tape is very useful for making bandages waterproof in the hoof area. The tape is also useful for covering poultices (Fig. 4.4).

Small sheep-size hoof clippers

These should be kept well oiled (Fig. 4.5).

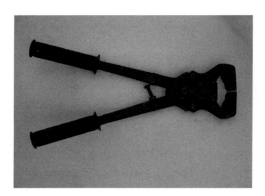

Fig. 4.3. Large hoof trimmers.

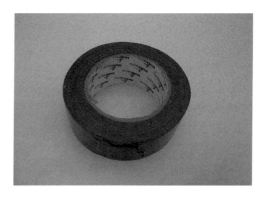

Fig. 4.4. Waterproof tape for bandaging feet. Often called gutter tape.

Equipment for Dentistry

Head light

There are some seriously bright torches available with heavy battery packs. These are not really required and a light which is easily taken on and off is preferable.

Large horse molar cutters

These are for detusking boars (Fig. 4.6).

Molar extraction forceps

Two pairs are required. They should be 20 cm long, one should be straight and the other should have the extracting jaws at right angles (Fig. 4.7).

Molar spreaders

A small pair 20 cm long is required (Fig. 4.8).

Mouth-washing syringe

A catheter tipped 60 ml syringe is adequate.

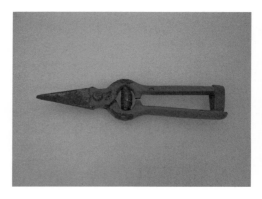

Fig. 4.5. Small sheep-size hoof clippers.

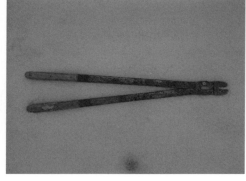

Fig. 4.6. Large horse molar cutters for cutting tusks.

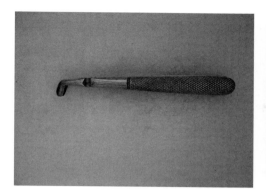

Fig. 4.7. 90° angle tooth extractors.

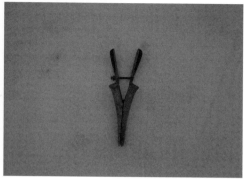

Fig. 4.9. A small vaginal speculum.

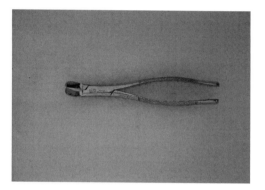

Fig. 4.8. Molar spreaders.

Small ruminant gag

These are hard to obtain. A suitable type is shown in Fig. 7.5.

Equipment for the Reproductive System

Vaginal speculum

These can be disposable and used with a head torch or a small hand torch. The small, stainless steel, duck-billed type affords the very best visibility (Fig. 4.9).

A dedicated box for Caesarean section

This should contain:

- 1 × 50 ml ketamine solution containing 100 mg/ml.
- 1 × 50 ml xylazine solution containing 100 mg/ml.
- 1 × 10 ml butophanol solution containing 10 mg/ml.
- 1 × 30 ml hard, non-disposable, plastic syringe.
- 1 × 5 cm 14 gauge needle.
- Sterile instruments including several 10 cm non-cutting and cutting curved suturing needles, one pair of needle holders, one pair of 'Gillies', one pair of rat-tooth dressing forceps, one pair of flat-ended dressing forceps, one scalpel blade holder, one large pair of straight scissors, four large pairs and two small pairs of artery forceps and two pairs of uterus-holding forceps.
- Scalpel blades which fit the scalpel blade holder in the sterile instruments.
- Polyglactin suture material.
- Monofilament nylon suture material.
- A sterile tray cloth.
- Navel clips.
- A sterile scrubbing brush.
- Two packets of large sterile swabs.
- Disposable syringes (10 ml and 20 ml).
- Disposable needles (4 cm × 18 gauge).
- Pieces of cotton wool in a bag for cleaning the skin.
- Bottle of surgical spirit.
- Bottle of chlorhexidine.
- 1 × 25 ml oxytocin injection containing 10 IU/ml.
- 1 × 100 ml water for injection.

- 1 × 5 mega-units of crystalline penicillin.
- 1 × 100 ml local anaesthetic.
- 100 ml aqueous suspension of a mixture of procaine penicillin and dihydro-streptomycin.

- Dopram drops.
- 100 ml bottle of an injectable non-steroidal anti-inflammatory drug (NSAID) licensed for pigs.
- An antibiotic aerosol.

5 Vaccines

Introduction

On large pig units vaccination plays a vital role in disease control. It is vital that the vaccines are used to the manufacturer's recommendations, particularly with regard to the age of the pig and the possibility of maternal passive immunity. It is also important that the risk of each disease is assessed and the vaccine is used only if actually required (see Table 5.1 below).

With pet pigs and small units assessing the need for vaccination is equally important. In the author's opinion, in the UK situation the only vaccine required by all pet pigs, and in fact all commercial pigs as well, is against *Erysipelothrix rhusiopathiae*.

There are fundamentally three types of vaccine:

- Live attenuated.
- Killed and inactivated.
- Small components of the pathogen.

When a non-infected animal is vaccinated there are three possible outcomes if the animal is then challenged by field infection (Brown, 2012):

- The animal's immune system is so strong it resists the infectious agent and the animal remains clean and healthy.
- The weight of infectious challenge is so high that, despite vaccination, the animal still succumbs to clinical disease.
- Immunity conferred by the vaccine is strong enough to resist clinical disease, but the pathogen is still able to enter the body and so the animal becomes a symptomless carrier of the pathogen. This is obviously most unsatisfactory as symptomless carriers remain undetected in the herd and can, under stressful situations, become excreters of the pathogen or even break down with clinical disease.

At the time of vaccination we cannot always be sure that the animal is not already infected. If a live vaccine is being used in such a circumstance then there is a risk of genetic recombination between the vaccinal strain and the field strain, thereby producing a new genetic variant of the pathogen which may or may not then be susceptible to the current vaccines. Volatile viruses, such as influenza virus, are changing genetically very frequently either as a result of straightforward mutations or as a result of recombination between various field strains.

PRRS virus also appears to mutate fairly regularly and the industry in the UK must

Table 5.1. Vaccines available.

Vaccine	Age of pig	Disease controlled	Importance	Extra details
Actinobacillus pleuropneumoniae	Growers	Acute respiratory disease caused by *A. pleuropneumoniae*	Very important when the disease is confirmed on a holding	No licensed vaccine in the UK but vaccine available elsewhere and can be made under licence in the UK
Atrophic rhinitis	Breeding animals to protect piglets	Rhinitis caused by *Pasteurella multocida* type D	This is important to protect weaners on infected farms	Not to be given unless the diagnosis is confirmed
Aujeszky's disease	Growers and breeders	To protect against all types of the disease	This is not justified in most countries	No licensed vaccine available in the UK
Chemical castration	Boars over 8 weeks of age	Boar taint, aggression and mounting behaviour	Only if slaughter is to be delayed	Not to be used in boars to be kept for breeding
Classical swine fever (CSF)	All pigs	To protect against all types of the disease	Very worthwhile in countries where the disease is endemic	Not licensed in the UK
Clostridial disease	Breeding animals to protect piglets and to protect breeding animals	Neonatal scour due to *Clostridium perfringens* and sudden death in adults due to *Clostridium novyi*	Very important in outdoor pigs. Rarely required in indoor pigs	A vaccine linked with an *E. coli* vaccine and a vaccine against clostridial disease on its own are both available in the UK
Escherichia coli	Breeding animals to protect piglets	Neonatal scour caused by *E. coli*	Extremely important if piglets are becoming infected	Often linked with clostridial vaccine. It is vital that the vaccine contains the correct K antigens
Erysipelas	All pigs over 6 weeks of age	All types of erysipelas	Vital for all pigs whether indoors or outdoors	Particularly important for smallholder pigs. Often linked with Parvo vaccination
Foot and mouth disease (FMD)	All pigs	The type of FMD to be covered should be chosen carefully	Unlikely to be permitted in most countries	Not licensed in the UK
Haemophilus parasuis	All pigs over 5 weeks of age	*H. parasuis*	Very important in herds where the disease occurs	Can be linked with enzootic disease vaccination

Table 5.1. Continued.

Vaccine	Age of pig	Disease controlled	Importance	Extra details
Lawsonia intracellularis	All pigs over 3 weeks of age	*L. intracellularis*	Important where the disease occurs	Is given in the drinking water
Mycoplasma hyopneumoniae	All pigs over 7 days of age	Enzootic pneumonia	Extremely important	Can be given with *H. parasuis* vaccination
Porcine circovirus	All pigs over 2 weeks of age	Post-weaning multisystemic wasting syndrome (PMWS)	Extremely important	Careful consideration needs to be given to the timing of the vaccination
Porcine parvovirus	Breeding animals to prevent reproductive problems	Parvovirus	Extremely important	Can be linked with erysipelas vaccination
Porcine reproductive and respiratory syndrome (PRRS)	Breeding animals to prevent reproductive problems	Prevent blue ear disease	Very important	Vaccines used should be regularly monitored as new strains emerge
Rotavirus	Breeding animals to protect piglets	Rotavirus	Only important in specific situations	There is a combined vaccine with TGE and *E. coli* but it is not licensed in the UK
Salmonella	For growing and fattening pigs	*Salmonella choleraesuis* and *Salmonella typhimurium*	Herd plan is much more important	Not available in the UK
Swine flu	All ages of pig over 8 weeks	Swine influenza A virus	Of limited use	Timing of vaccination is important
Tetanus toxoid	All ages of pig over 3 months of age	Tetanus	Normally not important in pigs	This should not be used as a routine but only when tetanus is a massive threat
Transmissible gastroenteritis (TGE)	Breeding animals to protect piglets	TGE	Not important in the UK	No licensed vaccine available in UK

remain alert to avoid importation of US strains and the so-called highly pathogenic strains.

When new variants occur, the available vaccines seldom give cross-protection. Potential new vaccines quite rightly have to undergo stringent testing and licensing procedures before marketing and so there is always a time lag between identification of a new pathogen or variant and widespread availability of a suitable vaccine.

The vast majority of vaccines administered to pigs are given by injection and so vaccines tend to be administered at times in the pig flow cycle when animals are handled or moved. At such times the dangers of operator self-injection are always present, particularly when large numbers of animals are being vaccinated. Self-injection of oil-based vaccines requires immediate medical attention.

Needles must be changed regularly to avoid sepsis not only at the site of injection in the pig but also if there is self-injection.

Vaccines to be given to Sows to Prevent Abortion

Erysipelothrix rhusiopathiae and porcine parvovirus

Pigs from 6 weeks of age should be given two injections, 4 weeks apart, of *E. rhusiopathiae* vaccine. A single injection of the combined vaccine should be given at least 2 weeks before mating. Then sows should receive a booster of the *E. rhusiopathiae* vaccine every 6 months, with the combined vaccine of *E. rhusiopathiae* plus porcine parvovirus (PPV) being given annually.

Porcine parvovirus

Gilts and young boars over 6 months of age should be given a single dose, 2 weeks before mating. Sows and boars require a booster dose annually.

Porcine reproductive and respiratory syndrome

For a primary vaccination course gilts require two injections 3–4 weeks apart, at least 3 weeks before mating. Sows require two injections 3–4 weeks apart. Vaccination of all sows in the herd within a short period is recommended. Revaccination is one injection at 60–70 days of each pregnancy, starting from the first pregnancy following the primary vaccination course.

Vaccines to be given to Sows to Give Passive Immunity to Neonatal Piglets

Introduction

The piglet is born with no bacterial flora in its intestine and potentially damaging organisms will begin to colonize the gut from birth onwards. Vaccines that are given to the sow or the gilt prior to farrowing aim to ensure colostral antibodies are well targeted to combat these organisms. Certain authorities advocate feedback attempts to work in a similar manner. However this is dangerous as other diseases may be spread inadvertently.

Atrophic rhinitis

A primary vaccination schedule is two injections separated by 6 weeks. Revaccination is one dose to be given to the sow ideally 2–6 weeks before farrowing.

Aujeszky's disease

Protection can be achieved by a single injection from the age of 14 weeks. Revaccination should be carried out on a herd basis every 4 months.

Clostridium tetani and *Clostridium perfringens* type B, C and D

Initially two injections with an interval of at least 3 weeks between injections, the second dose to be administered at least 3 weeks before farrowing, are required. Only a single booster dose is required in subsequent pregnancies at approximately 3–4 weeks pre-farrowing.

Escherichia coli (K99 strains) and *Clostridium perfringens* type B, C and D

A primary vaccination scheme consists of an initial course of two doses. The first dose should be given at service or, if necessary, at any time up to 6 weeks before farrowing. The second dose should be given 2 weeks before farrowing is expected. For a revaccination scheme a single dose should be given 2 weeks before farrowing is expected.

Escherichia coli (K99 strains)

A primary course of vaccination consists of two doses. The first injection should be given 5–7 weeks before farrowing and the second injection, 2 weeks before farrowing. Revaccination consists of a single injection 2 weeks before each subsequent farrowing.

Porcine circovirus type 2

Basic vaccination for gilts consists of two injections. The first injection should be followed in 3–4 weeks by the second injection, at least 2 weeks before mating. One further injection must be given, at least 2 weeks before farrowing. With sows the first injection should be followed in 3–4 weeks by a second injection, at least 2 weeks before farrowing. Revaccination consists of a single injection at each gestation, at least 2–4 weeks before farrowing.

Rotavirus, transmissible gastroenteritis and colibacillosis

There is a combined vaccine available but it is not licensed in the UK.

Swine influenza A virus

Primary vaccination consists of two injections of one dose from the age of 96 days, with an interval of 3 weeks between injections. A booster is possible at each stage of pregnancy and lactation. When vaccination is performed 14 days prior to farrowing with one dose, it provides maternally derived immunity to the piglets, which protects them from clinical signs of influenza at least until day 33 after birth.

Vaccines to be given to Growing and Fattening Pigs

Actinobacillus pleuropneumoniae

There is a vaccine available for serotypes 1, 5 and 7. It is not licensed in the UK.

Aujeszky's disease

An initial dose at 10 weeks of age should be followed by a second injection 2 weeks later.

Erysipelothrix rhusiopathiae

Pigs from 6 weeks of age should be given two injections 4 weeks apart.

Haemophilus parasuis

Vaccination is available for pigs at least 5 weeks of age. Two doses should be given separated by 2 weeks. Immunity will last for 14 weeks.

Lawsonia intracellularis

Administration of a single 2 ml dose orally to pigs from 3 weeks of age should be given irrespective of body weight. Vaccination is via the drinking water.

Mycoplasma hyopneumoniae

A single injection to be given between 3 and 10 weeks of age. Certain vaccines can be given as early as 7 days, but the majority of these require two doses 2–4 weeks apart.

M. hyopneumoniae and H. parasuis combined

Pigs are to be vaccinated from 7 days of age, with a second dose being given 14–21 days later.

Porcine circovirus type 2

A single injection from 2 weeks of age will give at least 17 weeks of immunity. Some vaccines claim to give immunity duration of 22 weeks.

Salmonella choleraesuis and Salmonella typhimurium

There is a live vaccine available but it is not licensed in the UK.

Streptococcus suis serotype 2

This bacterin is not licensed in the UK.

Swine influenza A virus

A primary course of vaccination consists of two injections of one dose: (i) from the age of 96 days, with an interval of 3 weeks between injections, to achieve duration of immunity over 6 months; or (ii) between the ages of 56 and 96 days, with an interval of 3 weeks between injections, to achieve duration of immunity over 4 months.

Tetanus

This should only be used in circumstances where there is an extra high risk of tetanus. Animals should be vaccinated when at least 3 months of age and given a second dose in 4–8 weeks. Revaccination should be carried out annually.

Improvac

A 2 ml dose contains a minimum of 300 μg of gonadotrophin-releasing hormone (GnRF) analogue-protein conjugate. It can be used in male pigs from 8 weeks of age to induce antibodies against GnRF to produce a temporary immunological suppression of testicular function (Fig. 5.1). It causes a reduction in entire male pigs after puberty of:

- Boar taint.
- Aggression.
- Mounting behaviour.

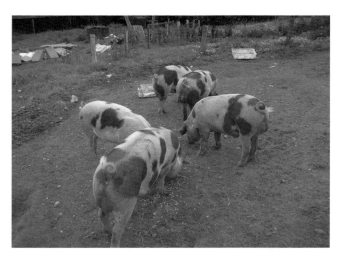

Fig. 5.1. These boars, which are late-maturing, require vaccination with a gonadotrophin-releasing hormone (GnRF) analogue-protein conjugate.

The onset of immunity can be expected 1 week after the second injection. Two doses of 2 ml should be given sc at least 4 weeks apart and at least 4–6 weeks before slaughter. There is in fact a zero meat withhold period. This vaccine should not be used in boars which are intended for breeding.

Vaccines to be given to Breeding Stock

Classical swine fever

There are inactivated and live vaccines to CSF available but none of them are licensed in the UK.

Erysipelothrix rhusiopathiae

Pigs from 6 weeks of age should be given two injections 4 weeks apart. Adult pigs should be revaccinated at 6-monthly intervals.

Foot and mouth disease

There are inactivated vaccines available for pigs but they are not licensed in the UK.

Table of Vaccines

Available vaccines are summarized in Table 5.1.

6 Sedation, Analgesia, Anaesthesia and Euthanasia

Sedation

Azaperone is the only sedative licensed for use in pigs in the UK. The dose is 2 mg/kg. It is not always very effective except when given im with 1 IU oxytocin/10 kg to gilts that are savaging their newborn piglets (Fig. 6.1). It is also licensed to prevent and cure fighting (including regrouping of piglets, porkers and fattening pigs): pigs from different litters or pens may be brought together into one pen immediately after administration. All animals should be treated. After a few minutes they lie down together for about 2 h, irrespective of their origin. Afterwards violent fights are unlikely to occur. During the time of treatment, untreated pigs should not be admitted to the pen. The product will not prevent aggressiveness in non-castrated adult boars. Newly weaned piglets may be treated together with other routine treatments on arrival at the fattening unit. Fighting animals become quiet shortly after the injection. The animals are unlikely to fight even after the effect of the drug has worn off. The drug is licensed to treat stress in the form of restlessness, anxiety, nervousness and excitation, e.g. because of pain: the dose for this between 1 and 2 mg/kg. The dosage should be adapted to the degree of excitation. If the animal is very nervous, the product may be given in divided doses at 15 min intervals.

Azaperone is licensed to transport boars: the animals should not be brought together within the first half hour following the injection because they are still likely to be aggressive; they should be left alone in a quiet environment during the induction period (approximately 30 min). The dose of 1 mg/kg should not be exceeded as a higher dose may cause the penis to be extruded, which may then be damaged. The drug may be used for transport of weaners at a dose of 0.4–2 mg/kg. It should be administered 15–30 min before transport to reduce mortality and weight loss during transport in order to prevent fighting. Animals should be given enough space to lie down. It is important to make sure there is adequate ventilation during transport. The drug may be used when there is cessation of parturition due to excitation, as an obstetric aid during normal delivery, inversion of the vagina, prolapse of the uterus or pathological straining. Azaperone may be used for premedication before local and general anaesthesia. The dose can be between 1 and 2 mg/kg. There are many indications: blood sampling, diagnostic examination, castration, prolapse of the rectum and wound treatment. Azaperone should not be used in the transportation or for regrouping of pigs which will be slaughtered prior to the end of the 10 day withdrawal period.

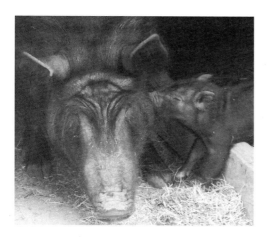

Fig. 6.1. Gilts may savage their piglets.

Analgesia

There are four useful injectable NSAIDs licensed for pigs in the UK: flunixin, ketoprofen, meloxicam and tolfenamic acid (see Appendix). They all follow similar pharmacokinetic pathways and therefore only a single drug needs to be carried by the ambulatory practitioner. Although these four NSAIDs are not licensed for oral use in pigs in the UK, they can be used under the cascade principle as the only licensed NSAID for oral administration is sodium salicylate, which has limited usage. Flunixin is available as a paste which can be given directly into a pig's mouth or in a sandwich of bread with chocolate spread. Flunixin is also available as granules. These can be sprinkled on the pig's food or once again put in a sandwich. Meloxicam is available as a liquid for oral administration to horses. This can easily be put on pig's food. Care should be taken with the dosage as the syringe supplied with the medication is calibrated for the weight of the horse. A dose needs to be worked out for a daily dose for the individual pig on a weight basis. For smaller pigs requiring analgesia with NSAIDs, tablets suitable for dogs, which are normally very palatable, can be given orally. This is allowed under the cascade principle.

Butorphanol is not licensed for pigs but may be used under the cascade principle. It is a very potent analgesic when given at 0.3 mg/kg by intramuscular injection. Unlike NSAIDs the analgesia lasts only for a maximum of 6 h.

Injectable ketoprofen given to sows suffering from postpartum dysgalactiae has been found to reduce pre-weaning piglet mortality. It is advisable that sows receive appropriate antibiotic treatment immediately after farrowing and that they also receive a single intramuscular injection of ketoprofen at 3 mg/kg.

Anaesthesia

Piglets

Anaesthesia is not well documented. However, masking very young piglets is quite easy with isoflurane or halothane without premedication. It should be remembered that certain pigs will possess a gene which makes them more susceptible to death from halothane anaesthesia. Owners should be made aware of this before it is used for anaesthesia. A signed disclaimer should be obtained from the owner.

Older growing pigs

The 15–25 kg weight range of pig can be masked down with isoflurane or halothane after premedication with azaperone at 2 mg/kg (Fig. 6.2). This will require good manual restraint for pigs in the heavier ranges. Unless this is available it is advisable to use a combination of drugs as described below for large growing pigs. It is advisable to weigh the pig accurately and obtain a signed disclaimer from the owner as such combinations are not licensed for pigs.

Large growing pigs and adults

A combination of drugs given im in the same hard, non-disposable syringe and a 14 gauge needle is the author's preference. The dose is 0.2 mg xylazine/kg, 10 mg ketamine/kg and 2 mg butorphanol/10 kg. It should be

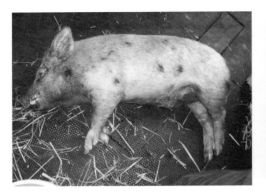

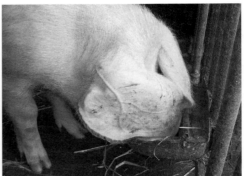

Fig. 6.2. A weaner pig under general anaesthetic (GA). **Fig. 6.3.** Veins on white ears are easier to visualize.

acknowledged that these products are not licensed for pigs in the UK either alone or in combination. This combination will give approximately 20 min of general anaesthesia, after a gentle induction which takes approximately 5 min. It also gives a slow gentle recovery. It is important that the pig is not stimulated during induction or recovery, but is allowed to lie quietly in lateral recumbency.

A 6% w/v pentobarbital solution at 1 ml/2.5 kg can be used to anaesthetize pigs by intravenous injection after premedication with azaperone at 2 mg/kg im. However this is not an easy technique. Although it is not licensed for pigs, the author has used a combination of azaperone at 2 mg/kg and acetylpromazine maleate at 0.1 mg/kg im. This will deepen the premedication and allow easier intravenous injection of the 6% w/v pentobarbitone. Veins on white ears are easier to visualize (Fig. 6.3).

Russian veterinary surgeons, after an intramuscular premedication with azaperone at 2 mg/kg and acetylpromazine maleate at 0.1 mg/kg, and butophanol at 2 mg/10 kg, inject pentobarbital at triple the normal dose directly into the testicle for castration. As soon as the pig is anaesthetized, castration is performed. Thus the source of anaesthetic is removed and the pig can be left to regain consciousness.

Epidural anaesthesia

This procedure is very hazardous, as the epidural space entered by the injecting needle in the lumbar area contains the lower spinal cord. The author has witnessed deaths from this procedure. The procedure can be used for the replacement of uterine, vaginal and rectal prolapses but is not recommended.

Euthanasia

Introduction

Euthanasia needs to be carried out in a variety of circumstances. Obviously if the pig is fit to travel from a welfare point of view and is suitable for human consumption, it should be transported to an abattoir. Veterinary surgeons are often asked to give advice on the fitness of a pig to travel. This may be an extremely difficult call. If in any doubt that there will be unnecessary suffering caused to the pig, the veterinary surgeon should advise euthanasia on-farm. If abattoirs require a 'certificate' this should be an 'owner's declaration' and not a certificate from a veterinary surgeon. A veterinary surgeon cannot certify that an animal on-farm is fit to be slaughtered at an abattoir as the practitioner does not know any medication that the pig may have received. Therefore any such certificate would breach the 'code of practice' laid down by the Royal College of Veterinary Surgeons.

If a pig is unfit to travel on welfare grounds, e.g. the animal having recently sustained a long-bone fracture, an on-farm slaughter for human consumption may be carried out under certain conditions.

There are two types of on-farm slaughter which are acceptable. Either the owner agrees that: (i) none of the pig is going to be sold and is only going to be eaten on-farm; or (ii) the pig is going to be slaughtered on-farm, then bled out and then transported in a hygienic manner to an abattoir within 1 h. If the meat is not going to be sold then a veterinary surgeon need not be involved.

Euthanasia may have to be performed by the pig keeper, who should be suitably trained, a knacker-man, who should have a licence, a licensed slaughterman or a veterinarian. It must be carried out humanely, with as little delay as possible. Movement to injured or ill animals should be kept to a minimum.

Euthanasia of piglets up to 5 kg

Euthanasia by trauma in baby pigs may be acceptable in a commercial situation and if performed correctly is within the welfare code, but is not acceptable for pet pigs. Unless moribund the piglet should be held by an assistant before being hit hard with a blunt instrument in the area of the brain. This is also not suitable if a PME of the brain is required.

For euthanasia of pet pigs up to 5 kg, they are best held on a sitting person's thighs with their head away from the handler. The handler holds the front legs firmly. The veterinary surgeon then stretches out the neck by pressure with one hand on the lower jaw. Then 5 ml of 20% w/v pentobarbitone sodium is injected into the anterior vena cava just cranial to the thoracic inlet. The 3 cm × 21 gauge needle is directed slightly medially and caudally. (The ear vein is very difficult to inject in small piglets).

In commercial or pet pigs a captive bolt may also be used. It should be directed at the point where the two lines from ear to opposite eye bisect on the head. It should be stressed that the pig should be held safely and securely when using such a method.

Euthanasia of pigs up to 15 kg

A captive bolt can be used on these pigs. It should be directed at the point where the two lines from ear to opposite eye bisect on the head. It should be stressed that the pig should be held safely and securely when using such a method.

Larger pigs and adults using a gun

These should be shot by a licensed knacker-man or slaughterman, or a veterinary surgeon, using a 0.32 calibre humane killer (Fig. 6.4) at

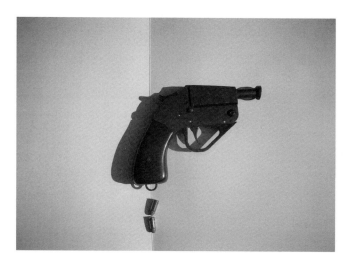

Fig. 6.4. A 0.32 calibre pistol for euthanasia of adult pigs.

the point where the two lines from ear to opposite eye bisect on the head. Often the pig will move if the firearm actually touches its head and therefore the clinician can stand directly in front of the pig and take very careful aim (Fig. 6.5). If a veterinary surgeon does not possess a firearms licence it is permitted to use a 12 bore shotgun, with permission of the licensed owner. The gun should be aimed from a distance of 10 to 50 cm away from the head into the same spot as described above.

Chemical euthanasia of pigs larger than 5 kg

This creates a real problem. Handling for intravenous injection is extremely difficult and injecting large volumes of fluid is also very difficult. In a quiet white pig it may be possible to use an ear vein, but this is extremely difficult in pigs with small ears such as Pot Bellied or Kunekune pigs of any age. It may be possible in lop-eared adults of other breeds to secure them with a nose snare and then inject into an ear vein.

In most pet pig situations the easiest protocol for adults is to give a GA im as described above. As soon as the pig is anaesthetized it should be given an injection of 50 ml of a solution containing 400 mg quinalbarbitone/ml and 25 mg cinchocaine hydrochloride/ml or 180 ml of a 6% w/v pentobarbital solution into the heart with a 10 cm spinal needle. Growing pigs can be given less on a pro rata basis.

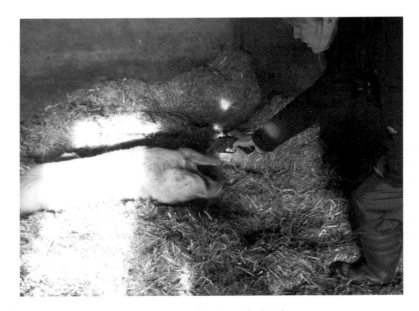

Fig. 6.5. Clinicians may take careful aim instead of touching the head.

7 Surgical Procedures

Surgical Procedures Related to the Skin

Abscesses

These are a sequel to: bites, burns, cuts or haematomas. Often the original cause is not apparent and they may even be a sequel to haematogenous spread of bacteria to a damaged area. A diagnosis should be established by cleaning the area and carrying out a paracentesis with a 14 gauge needle. If pus is found in the needle the diagnosis is confirmed. It is very important that practitioners do not lance a haematoma, granuloma or a tumour.

Abscesses need to be drained with a bold incision large enough to allow digital palpation of the inside of the abscess after washing out any diseased contents with warm saline. Antibiotics should be given with regard to meat withhold times in pigs near to slaughter weights.

Bites

These are caused by:

- Fighting between sows. Wounds often occur on the vulva.
- Fighting between boars. Wounds will be deep and occur on the body.
- Over-aggressive sexual foreplay by boars.
- Biting of nipples by piglets.
- Fighting between piglets. Wounds which occur on the face become infected.

Bites should be treated with injectable antibiotics which can be continued with water medication. If bites are severe, pigs should receive injectable NSAIDs which may be continued with water medication. Bites should be treated locally with either topical application of antibiotic sprays or with oily cream containing acriflavin and benzene hexachloride (BHC). Bites however severe should not be sutured because they will be contaminated, the sutures will break down and healing will be delayed.

Burns

These are caused by direct heat from heat lamps which have been positioned wrongly too close to the pigs. Heat lamps should always be secured with chain, not bailer twine, to prevent actual fires, which can be devastating in pig accommodation.

White pigs may become sunburnt. This should be avoided by always supplying shade and wallows. Burns should be treated with injectable antibiotics which can be continued with water medication. If burns are severe, pigs should receive injectable NSAIDs which may be continued with water medication. Burns should be treated topically with an oily cream containing acriflavin and BHC. If burns are too extensive, i.e. the burnt area is greater than 20% of the pig's total surface area, euthanasia should be carried out promptly. Sunburnt pigs should be treated topically with an oily cream containing acriflavin and BHC. In severe cases NSAIDs should be given.

Cuts

These are often caused by sharp edges of metal on damaged gates. Boars may cut sows or other boars with their tusks. These can be removed (see below). Cut pigs should receive injectable antibiotics which can be continued with water medication. They should also receive injectable NSAIDs. Depending on the severity of the wound these can be continued with water medication. As a general rule cuts should not be sutured unless they are very large as pigs heal very well by second intention. If suturing is to be attempted then a GA is recommended. Cuts can be covered by topical antibiotic sprays or with an oily cream containing acriflavin and BHC.

Haematomas

These normally occur in the ears of lop-eared breeds as a result of continuous shaking of the head, which is caused by mange mites. It is very important that the underlying cause, i.e. the mange, should be treated with injectable ivermectins. Pigs with haematomas should receive injectable antibiotics which can be continued with water medication and injectable NSAIDs, which also can be continued with water medication. Ear cleansers prepared for dogs can be instilled into the ears. Draining the haematoma is not recommended as the haemorrhage will be profuse. Full aseptic surgery under GA could be attempted but is not recommended, as healing will occur with time without surgery, leaving a not painful 'cauliflower ear'.

Neoplasia

Skin tumours are rare in pigs. The need to remove them would not be justified in a commercial situation. Owners may request their removal from pet pigs. The tumour and the drainage lymph nodes should be examined before surgery is agreed. If there is any evidence of metastatic spread then surgery should be declined on welfare grounds. If surgery is carried out then the tumour with a good margin should be removed under GA. A slice of the tumour and normal skin should be sent for histological examination.

Surgical Procedures Related to the Locomotory System

Acute lameness

Abscess in the foot

This is the most common cause of acute lameness in adult animals (Fig. 7.1). It may readily become a chronic condition (see below). Prompt aggressive antibiotic treatment is required. Poulticing the affected digit is worthwhile (Fig. 7.2). Pain relief with NSAIDs is mandatory.

Arthrogryposis

Arthrogryposis can cause acute lameness in baby pigs. Welfare is paramount and so

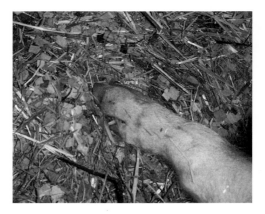

Fig. 7.1. A hoof abscess about to break out at the coronary band.

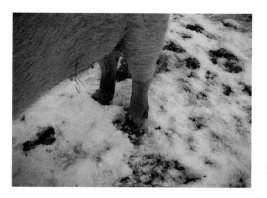

Fig. 7.2. An abscess on the left medial claw.

euthanasia is normally the correct course of action as such joints will not repair and will cause constant pain.

Benign enzootic paresis

This condition is part of the Teschen/Talfan disease syndrome (see Chapters 11 and 14). Pigs may show acute lameness.

Biotin deficiency

Pigs suffering from this deficiency will have damaged or weakened horn tissue in the soles of their feet and hence the most important presenting sign is lameness.

Erysipelas

Erysipelas rhusiopathiae can affect the joints and cause acute lameness.

Fractures

If fractures are below the knee or the hock in pet pigs they can be cast but normally euthanasia is indicated. If they are above the elbow or stifle euthanasia should always be carried out.

Foot and mouth disease

The most obvious sign of this disease is lameness (see Chapter 13).

Haemophilus arthritis

Haemophilus spp. will invade the joints of growing pigs and cause lameness. This will start as an acute lameness and unless treated aggressively will become chronic. Oxytetracycline is the antibiotic of choice, supported by a NSAID (see Chapter 9).

Infectious mycoplasma

Acute lameness is caused by *Mycoplasma hyorhinitis* and *Mycoplasma hyosynoviae*. These should be treated with tylosin or oxytetracycline by injection; both of these antibiotics can be given as a follow-up by water medication.

Osteochondrosis and epiphysiolysis

These are painful conditions in pigs causing acute lameness and should be treated with NSAIDs. Clinicians should reassess cases after treatment to make sure there has been an improvement. If there has been no improvement euthanasia should be carried out.

Osteomalacia

This would be thought to be a chronic condition but often the condition is manifest as an acute lameness. It may even account for sudden death. The bones become very weak from problems with calcium, phosphorus and vitamin D. There may be spontaneous fractures resulting in damage to a main artery, e.g. the femoral artery.

Slipped epiphysis of the femoral head

This is a condition mainly seen in young boars. The aetiology is unknown but it may be the result of osteochondritis. Euthanasia is recommended.

Splay leg

This is a condition of newborn piglets of unknown aetiology. If the piglets can manage to reach a teat, normally they will survive and improve slowly. If not then euthanasia is indicated.

Streptococcal arthritis

Streptococcus suis type 1 will cause fibrinous polyarthritis in piglets between 3 and 6 weeks old. They will show neurological signs of shaking, ataxia and recumbency. Equally they may just show signs of general malaise, some lameness and respiratory signs.

Chronic lameness

Arthrosis deformans

This is a condition of boars. The deformity of a joint will cause chronic lameness. Welfare is an issue. If practitioners are in any doubt the animal should be destroyed.

Bursitis

Obviously any inflammation in a bursa will potentially cause lameness. The most common to be affected in the adult pig is the bicipital bursa on the point of the shoulder. This normally occurs as a result of trauma from an animal trying to rush through a narrow opening. Lameness may well last for 6 weeks. NSAIDs are helpful.

Chronic septic arthritis

This can be caused by a very wide variety of arthritis pathogens. The best treatment is with high doses of antibiotics backed up with NSAIDs. It is important that the correct antibiotic is used from the efficacy standpoint. If there is no improvement the antibiotic should be changed. A prolonged course is likely to be necessary.

Heel ulceration

Hoof abscesses are painful and a difficult condition to treat. They may be due to sand cracks or they may have no obvious aetiology.

Drainage should be established if possible. If not a gauze dressing impregnated with magnesium sulfate poultice should be applied. This should be covered by waterproof gutter tape and kept on for several days. The animal should be treated with antibiotics and NSAIDs. If drainage has been established the poultice can be removed, but if not a new poultice should be applied. If the infection has tracked into the distal phalangeal joint normally euthanasia should be advised. In rare cases with much loved pet pigs, removal of the affected digit can be carried out. The pig should be given a GA (see Chapter 6). The leg should be thoroughly cleaned and a tourniquet applied above either the tarsus or the carpus. Embryotomy wire should be placed between the digits at an angle so that when the cut is complete the second phalanx of the affected digit is cut in half. With rapid sawing movement the diseased digit should be removed. The stump of the wound should be covered with a suitable antibiotic-impregnated dressing and the whole foot bandaged up. The bandage should then be covered with several layers of gutter tape. The pig should receive antibiotics and NSAIDs by injection. These should be continued for 10 days by water soluble medication. The bandage should be changed at weekly intervals until a clean granulation bed is totally covering the bony stump. Topical antibiotic spray can then be continued until total healing is accomplished.

Laminitis

Pigs do not actually get laminitis. Very fast-growing heavy hogs may get a coritis which will look like laminitis in that all four feet will be hot and painful. The amount of food should be reduced and they should be given NSAIDs. Care should be taken to stick to the meat withhold times.

Ligamental damage

Obviously some ligamental damage will cause severe lameness. Treatment with NSAIDs can be tried but if there is no response, euthanasia is indicated.

Overgrown hooves

This is a condition of backyard pigs of poor genetic conformation which do not receive sufficient exercise on a concrete surface (Fig. 7.3). Normally they can be trimmed without sedation in a pig crate. Old boars can have their feet trimmed while they are serving a sow.

Tarsitis

This is a specific condition of heavy sows or boars kept on concrete with insufficient bedding. It used to be very common when sows were kept in tethers. The animal must be given a soft bed and NSAIDs. Antibiotics are only required if there is sepsis.

Hoof trimming

This is very rarely required in commercial pigs. However with pet pigs claws will become overgrown (Fig. 7.3). Often the cause of this is poor genetic conformation rather than lack of movement on an abrasive surface, e.g. concrete.

Recumbency

This is particularly common in pigs which have been bred for a long back to increase

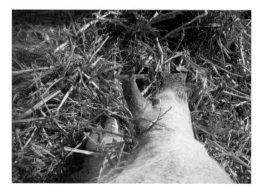

Fig. 7.3. A claw in need of trimming.

bacon production. Recumbency can be caused by a space-occupying lesion in the vertebral canal, e.g. an abscess, a haematoma or a tumour (Fig. 7.4). Treatment with antibiotics and NSAIDs can be tried but if unsuccessful euthanasia is indicated. Fractured vertebrae will cause recumbency but they are extremely rare in pigs. Euthanasia is indicated. Trauma to the back or pelvis at mating or from fighting is common. NSAIDs can be tried but if not successful euthanasia is indicated.

Surgical Procedures Related to the Gastroenteric System

Atresia ani

This is an inherited defect which will be observed soon after birth. Careful examination should be carried out to differentiate this condition from atresia coli. These cases should be destroyed. To treat atresia ani, the area below the tail should be cleaned carefully. A small bleep of local anaesthetic should be placed over the bulge formed by the backlog of faeces. A small stab cruciate incision should be made to allow the free passage of faeces. The pig should be re-examined in 3 days to confirm the passage of faeces. It is prudent on the day of surgery to carefully examine all the other piglets in the litter.

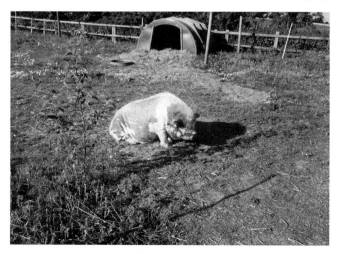

Fig. 7.4. A pig unable to rise.

Atresia ani may be present in other litter-mates that will require similar surgery. All of the pigs in the litter should be identified so that they go for slaughter and are not kept for breeding.

Gastric torsion

This can occur in adult pigs after feeding. The pig will be found either dead or bloated and *in extremis*. Splenic torsion may also occur, adding to the shock. If pigs appear bloated, forced exercise has been suggested. However, in the author's experience this has not been successful. It is therefore a welfare issue and euthanasia should be carried out promptly.

Gastric ulceration

This is known to occur with serious diseases like SF and salmonellosis. It can also occur with transmissible gastroenteritis (TGE) in adults, which show very mild signs of the dis-ease but are left with gastric ulcers as a sequel. There has been a link with *Helicobacter pylori* postulated as a cause for gastric ulcers but this has never been proven. The animals with gastric ulceration will have black tarry faeces. Treatment with 4 mg omeprazole daily per rectum has been suggested. There has been no evidence shown of its effectiveness.

Intestinal obstruction

Intestinal obstruction has a variety of causes and can occur in all ages of pig. Some causes will be linked with certain ages of pig and certain types of husbandry. The most com-mon cause of intestinal obstruction in adult pigs kept outside is the ingestion of foreign bodies, normally stones. Intussusception of the small intestine can occur in any age of pig but is more common in pigs less than 30 kg. Intestinal volvulus tends to be more common in adult pigs. Intestine trapped in an inguinal hernia is extremely rare. Normally pigs will behave completely like their littermates even

with quite large inguinal hernias. Unlike in stallions, prolapse and strangulation through an inguinal hernia has never been witnessed by the author. Umbilical hernias are a common inherited condition in pigs. Trapped small intestine has only been seen once by the author. It was in a 20 kg Landrace gilt pig. The intestine was irreparably damaged and the pig was promptly destroyed.

The normal clinical signs of intestinal obstruction are: lethargy, anorexia, a subnor-mal rectal temperature, a tacky feel as the thermometer is withdrawn and cold ears. If small intestine is trapped in a hernia there will be pain and swelling in the area of the hernia.

Further diagnostics could include ultra-sonography and radiography. These are unlikely to be requested except in pet pigs. Ultrasonography should be carried out trans-abdominally. It may need to be repeated after 12–24 h as the presence of stones needs to be assessed carefully. Some stones present in the stomach are not likely to be significant. It is their presence in the small intestine which is important. Ultrasonography might be helpful with diagnosis of trapped intestines in hernias to check for intestinal movement. Lack of movement would indicate bowel compromise and therefore euthanasia can then be carried out without delay. Radiography is only likely to be helpful in small pigs and would require a GA. The significance of abdominal foreign bodies will be difficult to interpret. Gassy loops of bowel will be diagnostic.

Treatment of intestinal obstruction caused by a foreign body, an intussusception or a volvulus should include antibiotics and NSAIDs. Some clinicians favour liquid paraf-fin. This should be poured into the only water source available to the pig. It will float on the top and so the pig will swallow some when-ever it drinks. Often this will help the stone to move down the small intestine, the pig will then show some clinical improvement and then it will stick again and the pig will deteri-orate again. As soon as the stone enters the large intestine there will be a marked clinical improvement. Liquid paraffin will also act as a diagnostic tool as its presence as a glinting cover to a stool will indicate patency of the bowel.

Abdominal surgery is outside the author's experience. It is feasible, certainly in smaller pigs. If a stone could be felt in the small intestine it could be removed or milked into the large intestine. At least with a laparotomy the extent of any disease process can be assessed so that euthanasia can be carried out promptly.

The treatment options for intestinal entrapment in an inguinal hernia will vary depending on the likelihood of the bowel being still viable, i.e. if there is pain in the area and the pig is not cold and shocked. Surgery in smaller pigs will be possible with local infiltration of local anaesthetic. Surgery in large boars will require a GA. The area should be cleaned with the pig held upside down or, in the case of large boars, with the hind quarters being raised. A careful incision should be made into the swollen scrotum without penetrating the tunics. If possible the intestine should be milked back into the abdomen. The testicle should then be the only organ within the tunic. Two pairs of large artery forceps should be placed side by side across the chord within the tunic. The proximal pair should be removed and a transfixing ligature of absorbable suture material should be applied in the groove left by the forceps. The testicle should be removed by a cut distal to the remaining pair of artery forceps. The skin should be closed with interrupted horizontal mattress sutures of monofilament nylon. If the pig is very shocked and it is likely that the bowel is no longer viable or if the bowel is viable but cannot be milked back into the abdomen, the tunics will have to be opened carefully. This is beyond the author's experience. However the bowel should be checked for viability. If it is viable the inguinal ring will have to be enlarged to allow its return. If it is not viable then bowel resection will need to be carried out. In both instances the testicle should be removed by an open method. In both instances an attempt will need to be made to close the inguinal ring before skin closure. Antibiotics and NSAIDS should be given in all cases.

Boars which have been castrated as adults need to be kept for a minimum of 2 months to lessen the boar taint before slaughter for human consumption.

The treatment of intestinal entrapment in an umbilical hernia will require a GA so that the pig can be put into dorsal recumbency. The hernia sack and the surrounding area should be surgically prepared. A careful incision should be made into the hernial sack and the bowel should be carefully examined for viability. If non-viable the affected part should be resected. The bowel will need to be restored by an end-to-end anastomosis. After carefully checking the suture line the bowel should be returned to the abdomen. Horizontal mattress sutures of monofilament nylon should be laid but not tightened across the abdominal defect, making sure that the peritoneal surfaces will be in apposition when the sutures are tightened. When the surgeon is totally happy that sufficient sutures have been laid, the sutures can be tightened individually. On no account should further sutures be laid once the abdomen is closed. The subcuticular tissue should be closed with a continuous layer of absorbable sutures. The skin should be closed with single horizontal mattress sutures of monofilament nylon. Antibiotics and NSAIDs should be given in all cases.

Prolapsed rectum in fattening pigs

This is caused by continuous violent coughing due to respiratory disease. It can be prevented by controlling the respiratory disease with vaccination and good husbandry. When it has occurred treatment of the underlying respiratory disease is vital. This is normally carried out with suitable antibiotics and NSAIDs.

There are two methods of surgical correction.

1. The conventional method requires the pig to be held upside down by its hind legs. The prolapsed rectum and surrounding area should be cleaned and local anaesthetic should be infiltrated around the anal ring. After a few minutes a purse-string suture of thick braided nylon should be laid around the anal ring but not tied. The prolapse should be replaced using lubricant. The suture should be tied so that only one finger could be introduced through the anal ring. The pig should be fed on a laxative diet or have liquid paraffin continuously put in its water. The suture should be removed in 14 days.

2. A possible method mainly for non-veterinarians requires a 10 cm length of rubber sprayer hose 2.5 cm in diameter with rubber ridges and a length of uterine tape. The pipe should be inserted with at least half its length into the anal ring inside the prolapse using plenty of lubricant. A length of uterine tape should be tied around the prolapse as close to the anal ring as possible in one of the rubber grooves. The pig should be given antibiotics and NSAIDs. The pig MUST be kept separate until the prolapse has rotted off and a new anal ring has been formed.

A rare sequel to this condition is rectal stricture. This condition can also occur in growing pigs without following a prolapsed rectum. The pig will appear to be bloated. On careful examination the scarring of the rectum will be seen. Only very small ribbons of faeces may be passed. In theory careful radical surgery would cure the condition. However humane destruction is normally indicated.

Prolapsed rectum in sows

Normally this condition occurs around parturition. It can be prevented by giving sows a laxative diet before parturition and for a few days after. There are two methods of surgical correction which are similar to those in fattening pigs but on a larger scale (see above). The sow needs to be restrained in a crate. The purse-string suture when tightened needs to be able to accommodate three fingers. If the method for non-veterinarians is used, the hosepipe needs to be 6 cm in diameter and 20 cm long.

Tooth problems

Before looking in a pig's mouth it is important that clinicians know what is normal.

A pig has a diphyodont dentition, i.e. a deciduous and a permanent set of teeth. There are 28 deciduous teeth. On one side there are three incisors on the maxilla and the mandible. There is one canine on the maxilla and the mandible. There are three premolars on the maxilla and the mandible. All 28 of these teeth are replaced and a pig also has another four premolars and 12 molars, so that a pig has 44 permanent teeth.

At birth a piglet has four incisors and four canines. Four more incisors erupt in 3 weeks and a further four in 3 months. During the first month 12 premolars erupt. The first permanent premolar and first molar erupt at approximately 5 months. The deciduous canine is replaced by the permanent canine before a pig is a year old. This is followed by the deciduous incisors which are replaced roughly during the second year of the pig's life. Three deciduous premolars are replaced in the second year of a pig's life. Two further molars also erupt at this time.

Tooth problems are rare in pigs except in very old backyard pigs. They will be manifest as a pig reluctant to eat nuts and spitting out other food. There will be malodorous breath. The pig needs to be examined carefully with a gag (Fig. 7.5) and a head torch under a GA (Fig. 7.6). Any rotten cheek teeth which are digitally loose (Fig. 7.7) should be removed (Fig. 7.8) with small equine molar extraction forceps. Antibiotics and NSAIDs should be given post-operatively. Owners should be instructed to monitor the pig carefully so that if the problem recurs,

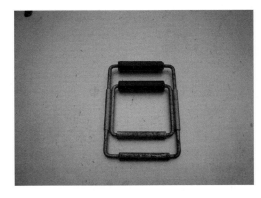

Fig. 7.5. A gag for pigs.

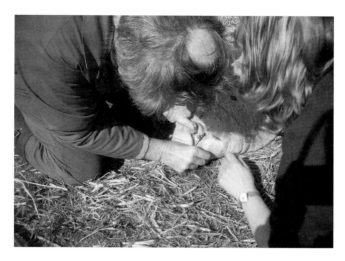

Fig. 7.6. A careful examination of the teeth under a general anaesthetic (GA).

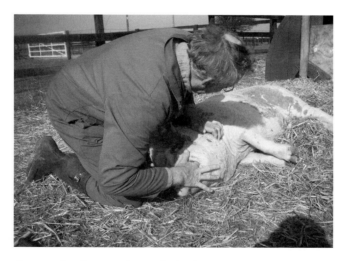

Fig. 7.7. Cheek tooth removal under general anaesthetic (GA).

which is likely, they must seek veterinary attention without delay.

Growing backyard pigs will rarely have problems with retained deciduous incisors. These will normally be shed eventually before the pig reaches 3 years of age. If they are retained after this age they extremely rarely cause problems for the pig. Removal is very difficult and should be avoided if possible. A GA is required and careful elevation of the deciduous incisor is time consuming. The tooth root must not be broken as it needs to be removed in its entirety.

Old boars will develop long, extremely sharp canines. These may be broken off by trauma but will not cause any problems. When they are left they are dangerous to pig handlers and also to other pigs. They do not have a pulp cavity above the gingival margin and so can be cut off at this point without causing pain or infection. Restraint is the main problem. One simple way is to cut them off while a boar is mounting a sow. Otherwise the boar should be restrained in a crate and held with a pig snare. The ideal method is with equine molar shears (Fig. 7.9).

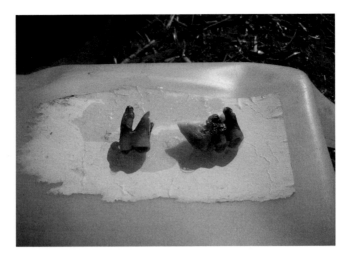

Fig. 7.8. Diseased teeth removed from a pig.

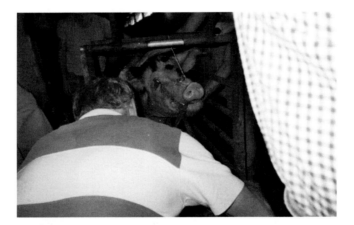

Fig. 7.9. Detusking a boar.

Embryotomy wire may be used but this will become very hot and will continually break. Because of the long length of time required the boar is liable to become fractious. Sedation with azaperone is not effective and a GA may be required. This increases the risk of the procedure.

Umbilical hernia

This is an inherited condition and therefore the parents of affected piglets should be recorded and if several piglets are affected they should not be bred from again but culled. Usually affected piglets in a commercial situation will be allowed to reach slaughter weight and may be sent to the abattoir as normal as there are usually no welfare implications. If the hernia is large and there is ulceration of the skin below the hernia, the pig should be slaughtered on-farm. In theory the carcass is fit for human consumption but in reality the difficulties with slaughtering and dressing out for a home kill are too onerous and so the carcass is normally sent off like any other cull.

The difficulty arises for the practitioner in the pet pig situation as owners naturally are reluctant to destroy the animal. Most small hernias will not cause problems and may be left alone. The author has only seen one pig with a strangulated bowel in an umbilical hernia. If the hernia is large then surgery is possible and should be attempted, after careful consultation with the owner, as soon as possible. Anaesthesia is much easier in baby pigs which can be masked down (see Chapter 6). The surgery is relatively straightforward and the technique is the same as for a dog. It requires care when stitching up the skin as piglets may interfere with the wound and therefore many small, single, interrupted sutures will be required. The pig should be kept away from its littermates for 10 days. In most pet pig situations it will be on its own or have just a single friend. It should be castrated at the same time if it is a male. On no account should the hernia be reduced and a rubber elastrator ring applied as pigs will chew the area and there is a danger of evisceration.

Surgical Procedures Related to the Urinary System

Preputial damage

The cause of this is unknown but it is likely to be related to sexual work as it tends to occur in groups of boars. The prepuce becomes very inflamed and necrotic. If caught in the early stages antibiotics and NSAIDs will be curative. If the prepuce is severely damaged and the local lymph nodes enlarged, surgical debridement will have to be carried out under GA.

Retroversion of the bladder

This can occur in sows at farrowing. The inverted bladder will feel like a 15 cm diameter ball blocking the vagina. It should be replaced with plenty of lubricant and the use of an equine nasogastric tube. It is not a difficult procedure. The piglets can then be drawn. Small doses of 5 IU of oxytocin should be given im at half-hourly intervals to aid parturition, which should be supervised. Only when parturition is complete may the

practitioner relax, knowing that the bladder will not retrovert again. The sow should be given antibiotics and NSAIDs. The sow should not be bred from again.

Surgical Procedures Related to the Reproductive System

Introduction to castration

With modern pig production methods using high-quality genetic stock and well-balanced diets, castration is unnecessary as pigs will reach slaughter weight before there is any real sexual activity and before there is any danger of the meat being rejected for boar taint. Therefore the vast proportion of pigs will not be castrated. This is good from a welfare point of view. If in a commercial situation it becomes apparent that pigs may become sexually mature before slaughter then they should be chemically castrated (see Chapter 5).

In certain different circumstances pigs will need to be castrated:

- Pet pigs.
- Pigs of slow-maturing breeds.
- Boars kept for breeding but found not suitable.
- Rescued pigs.

With pet pigs and pigs of slow-maturing breeds it is important that pigs are castrated as young as possible, i.e. 2 weeks of age. Owners should be instructed accordingly.

Castration

Before attempting castration it is vital that a check is made for the presence of an inguinal hernia. This condition is inherited, so in a commercial situation any boar siring affected piglets should be culled. Because of inbreeding this condition is particularly common in pot-bellied pigs.

Normal castration in piglets under 2 months of age is straightforward. Anaesthesia is not required, although pet pig owners may demand it. It is prudent to remove the piglets out of earshot not only from the sow but also the owner. The noise made by the piglets is related more to the handling rather than to the pain of the procedure. The pig is held by the hocks with its belly facing an assistant, who grips the chest of the pig between his or her knees. The scrotum is cleaned. A testicle is squeezed into the scrotum and a bold incision is made through the skin and the tunics so the testicle pops out. The testicle and the cord are twisted and pulled quickly out (Fig. 7.10). The process is repeated for the other testicle and the area is sprayed with antibiotic spray.

Castration in piglets under 2 months of age with an inguinal hernia requires much more controlled surgery. The pig is held by the hocks with its belly facing an assistant, who grips the chest of the pig between his or her knees. The scrotum is cleaned. A testicle is squeezed into the scrotum and a careful incision is made through the skin but not through the tunics. Using blunt dissection the testicle is brought through the incision with its tunics intact and any abdominal contents are milked back into the abdomen. Normally the abdominal contents have fallen back into the abdomen on account of gravity. A pair of artery forceps is placed across the chord. A transfixing ligature of absorbable material is placed proximal to the artery forceps. The testicle is removed distal to the pair of artery forceps with a scalpel

cut. The artery forceps are then carefully removed. A single horizontal mattress suture is placed in the skin. The process is repeated for the second testicle and the area is sprayed with antibiotic spray.

Castration of larger boars will require a GA. The surgery is the same but on a larger scale (see above). There is no need to use any emasculators however large the boar.

Vasectomy

The need for this surgical procedure in commercial pigs is limited. It is not appropriate in pet pigs as castration is normally indicated. A GA is required and the pig is placed in dorsal recumbency. Full aseptic precautions should be taken. The pig should be injected with antibiotics and NSAIDs before starting the surgery. A 4 cm incision should be made just cranial to the testicle. The spermatic cord should be exteriorized by blunt dissection. It should then be anchored by inserting a pair of artery forceps below it. Care should be taken not to exteriorize the penis. The spermatic cord should be palpated on the medial aspect to find the vas deferens which will be felt as a tubular structure (similar to the plastic holding the ink in a ballpoint pen). A small incision should be

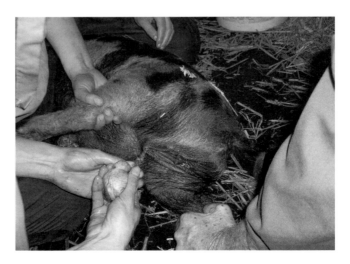

Fig. 7.10. The testicle is twisted before pulling.

made into the cord over the vas deferens, taking care not to cause haemorrhage in the many blood vessels beside it. A 2.5 cm length of vas deferens should be pulled out and clamped at both ends with a pair of artery forceps. Ligatures of absorbable suture material should be placed below both pairs of forceps. The section of the vas deferens bounded by the two pairs of artery forceps should be removed and placed in a small container of formal saline. Two sutures should be placed in the skin after removal of the artery forceps and replacement of the

cord. The procedure should be repeated on the other side.

The container holding the two pieces of vas deferens should be carefully labelled with the date, the owner's name and the pig's number. If the practitioner is satisfied that he has removed two sections of vas deferens the sample can be stored as there is no need for any histological examination. If the practitioner has any doubts the sample should be sent to a laboratory for confirmation that two pieces of vas deferens have been removed.

8 Diseases of the Gastroenteric System

Introduction

The predominant signs, i.e. diarrhoea, anorexia, pyrexia, vomiting, dysentery and tenesmus, make the clinical diagnosis of gastroenteric disease fairly straightforward. The clinician will find the age of the pig and any other history, e.g. an alteration to diet, helpful in trying to establish causality. Faeces samples rather than rectal swabs, which are not normally sufficient, are likely to be vital. The ultimate mode of diagnosis may have to be a series of post-mortems.

Mode of Infection

Many enteric organisms and parasites are very resistant to desiccation and disinfection, particularly if this does not follow thorough cleaning. Pet or smallholder pigs are likely to become infected by faeces on visitors' boots. Because of this, commercial pig-men, however well meaning, should be kept away from backyard pigs. Commercial pigs are particularly vulnerable to incoming stock and transport lorries. These lorries may include those delivering feed or bedding. They may be vehicles collecting dead stock. The lorries may be collecting pigs for sale; weaners, fatteners or cull sows and boars may also be a risk. All transport lorries should stay outside the farm gates and be loaded and unloaded there.

Prevention

Pig farms should avoid bringing live pigs on to the farm. The advantages of having a closed herd are many. For fattening herds, having an 'all-in all-out' policy is vital. All outgoing pigs should be taken and loaded outside the perimeter in special facilities. Equally, all dead pigs should be either incinerated on-farm or taken outside the perimeter for collection. All visitors have to be 'pig free' for 3 days before entry. All visitors should wear boots and overalls provided by the farm at the gates (veterinarians particularly should remember to uphold strict biosecurity). All visitors should leave their vehicle outside the farm gates. A visitors' book should be kept recording all visitors' names. The company or practice they work for should be recorded, as well as the last pig farm they have visited and the date of that visit. The reason for the visit should be noted. Pig farmers should try to limit the number of visits by outsiders to a minimum.

Causes of Enteric Disease

These are: viruses, bacteria, protozoa, endoparasites, poisoning, changes of nutrition (as a rule of thumb, epidemic enteric disease is seen less in backyard pigs than in commercial pigs but problems with nutrition are more common in backyard pigs) and other miscellaneous causes.

Enteric Diseases Caused by Viruses and Their Treatment

Epidemic diarrhoea

This is caused by a coronavirus. The disease is also called porcine epidemic diarrhoea (PED). It shows clinical signs very similar to TGE (see below). Both conditions are now rare but TGE was common in the UK in the 1960s. Epidemic diarrhoea was first recorded in the UK in 1972. Historically it was less common than TGE. There are two forms of the disease. Both have a high morbidity like TGE but a reduced mortality. One type occurs in piglets less than 5 weeks old. It causes profuse watery diarrhoea. Some young piglets may vomit. The only sign seen in older pigs is a transitory anorexia with evidence of abdominal pain. The second type causes diarrhoea in the entire herd with a few deaths in the neonatal piglets. The two types can only be differentiated on clinical signs. However there is a specific monoclonal antibody test available to differentiate epidemic diarrhoea from TGE. There is no specific treatment available. Extra warmth and the provision of electrolytes are helpful. There is no vaccine available.

Rotavirus infection

This is a very common condition in baby pigs. Rotaviruses occur in many species of farmed livestock, including birds. The rotavirus which normally infects piglets is from the Group A type of viruses. Groups B, C and E are also found. The virus is very stable and can survive in the environment for several months. When the virus infects very young piglets there is a high morbidity and a high mortality. The piglets are depressed, anorexic and reluctant to move. They may vomit. These signs are followed by profuse yellow diarrhoea. This will continue for a few days. The piglets will become less ill quite soon

provided they are kept warm. The diarrhoea may continue for up to 2 weeks. However if piglets are over 1 week of age when they contract the disease, the mortality is much reduced particularly if there is good temperature control and electrolytes are provided. Older pigs are more resistant and often the disease is subclinical. It is usually only found in conjunction with another pathogen. Some authorities advise removing the diarrhoeic piglets from the sow. In the author's experience this is not worthwhile, as the piglets become weak and die. Antibiotics and antiprotozoal drugs should be given if there is evidence of concurrent infections. Diagnosis is by isolation of the virus in a faeces sample using electron microscopy and a fluorescent antibody test (FAT). Antigens and antibodies can be confirmed with an enzyme-linked immunosorbent assay (ELISA). Serology of a few of the herd will confirm the disease retrospectively. A post-mortem will show a typical milk-filled intestine with dehydration. Histology of the small intestine will show villous atrophy. The disease spreads relatively slowly. An 'all-in all-out' regime in the farrowing houses is well worthwhile with thorough cleaning and disinfection. There is no vaccine available.

Transmissible gastroenteritis

This highly contagious disease is caused by a coronavirus. There has not been a major outbreak in the UK for over 30 years. The incidence of the virus is very low on mainland Europe. The disease is widespread in the USA. The virus which causes TGE is very similar to the virus which causes PED (see above). It may be that there is some crossimmunity so that low levels of PED virus prevent widespread TGE.

In a naive herd which has no previous exposure to either TGE or epidemic diarrhoea, an outbreak of TGE is explosive. The incubation period is 2 days. There is almost 100% morbidity, with 100% mortality in baby pigs but few or no symptoms in adults. Baby piglets will vomit and have characteristic, watery, foul-smelling, greenish yellow diarrhoea. This is followed by severe dehydration, collapse and death. If diarrhoea occurs in the adults it is short-lived. It is important that they have ample access to clean fresh water. Electrolytes may be helpful. Death is so rapid in baby piglets that it normally occurs before euthanasia can be carried out. Infected pregnant sows will pass on immunity to their piglets so that the disease will appear to have run its course. Sadly the immunity seems to be short-lived, so another outbreak is likely to occur in 6 to 9 months. Diagnosis is based on virus isolation by FAT on a faeces sample. There is an ELISA and a specific monoclonal antibody test available. On post-mortem the piglets will be in a very poor dehydrated condition. Their stomachs will be empty. There will be the greenish yellow fluid in their intestines. As there is no treatment but immunity is rapidly established in a herd and there is no vaccine available, it is suggested that dung from infected piglets is given to in-pig sows to establish immunity which can then be passed on as passive immunity to the piglets. Such procedures are not without hazard and so should be given very careful consideration. The disease is really a disease of large commercial herds. It is only likely to attack the small pig herd which is buying in gilts.

Vomiting wasting disease

This disease is caused by a coronavirus, the haemagglutinating encephalomyelitis virus. It was first recorded in Canada in 1962. It occurs in the UK; clinical signs are rare although serological studies indicate that the virus is very widespread. The virus is spread by the oro-nasal route. The incubation period is within 3–5 days. It affects piglets between 5 and 20 days of age. As the name suggests, they vomit, slowly lose weight and die. They have a raised rectal temperature and are constipated. They are depressed and anorexic. A very few piglets may show neurological signs of ataxia and difficulty in swallowing. Not all the piglets in a litter will be affected. The healthy piglets will look very different from the poor wasted infected piglets, which will often be very hairy. Sows rarely show any clinical signs except a brief fever and anorexia for 12 h. Gross post-mortem findings are not

helpful. Twenty-five per cent of cases will show an encephalomyelitis on CNS histopathology. There is some colostral immunity. The bigger pigs will get an active immunity. This is not a disease of outdoor pigs as the virus is readily killed by ultraviolet light. Diagnosis is by virus isolation or FAT on the faeces. A retrospective diagnosis can be made with serology. There is no treatment and euthanasia is indicated. There is no vaccine available. Passive colostral immunity will protect the piglets from disease.

Enteric Diseases Caused by Bacteria and Their Treatment

Campylobacter enteritis

This is a complex condition as *Campylobacter* spp. are ubiquitous but rarely are clinical signs linked to the presence of an organism. The main organism is *Campylobacter coli* but other *Campylobacter* spp., e.g. *C. jejuni*, *C. hyointestinalis* subsp. *hyointestinalis* or subsp. *lawsonii*, *C. mucosalis*, *C. hyoilei*, *C. lari* or *C. lanienae*, may be involved. *Campylobacter* spp. classically cause a mucoid creamy diarrhoea or even dysentery in piglets less than 3 weeks of age. They will also cause mucoid diarrhoea in weaned piglets which are not immune.

In piglets the incubation period is 3 days. They will have a slight rise in rectal temperature before the diarrhoea, which will continue for a few days. There is a sharp loss of condition but death is rare. Piglets contract the infection from sows. Some will then become carriers. Therefore diagnosis can only be confirmed if there is a definite profuse growth of the organism or from a post-mortem showing massive enlargement of the lymphoid tissue in the terminal ileum. Neomycin or tetracyclines are the preferred antibiotics given by the oral route.

Clostridial diarrhoea

This is quite common in outdoor pigs not only in the UK but also elsewhere in the world. It can be caused by *Clostridium perfringens* type A or C. Type A is less severe than type C;

the latter causes 100% mortality in piglets less than a week old. The faeces are claret coloured. The hind quarters of the piglets will become covered in bloody faeces. This is almost a pathognomonic sign. Confirmation of the diagnosis relies on mouse protection toxin tests which should be avoided if possible. PME will be helpful. The jejuni of infected piglets will be extremely inflamed and filled with blood-stained contents. Rarely pigs may survive type C infection but will be stunted. At that stage euthanasia should be strongly advised. Type A does not cause the haemorrhagic diarrhoea but slightly less acute, yellow pasty diarrhoea. PME will reveal necrotic areas in the small bowel but no haemorrhage. Control is labour intensive as the organism is ubiquitous. Antibiotics are effective but not really appropriate. Susceptible pigs can be given hyperimmune antiserum at birth. The best course of action is to vaccinate the sows with the correct clostridial vaccine 2 weeks before farrowing.

There are other *Clostridium* spp. which cause enteric problems in pigs. *Clostridium difficile* has been isolated from pigs and shown to cause acute haemorrhagic diarrhoea or a more chronic scouring. These isolates have been found in North America and France but not in the UK. Both A and B toxins have been found. It must be remembered that the organism is zoonotic. In piglets under 1 week of age it causes abdominal distension followed by diarrhoea. There is marked dehydration with sunken eyes. There is scrotal oedema. This unusual sign is pathognomonic for the condition. These animals will not recover and should be euthanased. There is both high morbidity and mortality. On post-mortem there is marked large bowel pathology but no small bowel pathology. This is another pathognomonic finding. Diagnosis with ELISA or polymerase chain reaction (PCR) can be made from the large bowel. Rarely mastitis has been reported in sows. Fluoroquinolones are suggested as treatment in sows. Treatment of piglets is rarely rewarding but tylosin has been suggested. There is no vaccine or antiserum available. Vancomycin and metronidazole are not licensed for pigs. They should not be used in pigs but should be reserved for human treatment.

Pigs will get tetanus caused by *Clostridium tetani*. It is extremely rare and in the normal course of pig husbandry, pigs do not require any preventive measures e.g. vaccination or antiserum. The one exception is when piglets, normally pet pigs, are castrated in a stable which has been used for horses. In these circumstances, it is advisable to give them 2 ml of tetanus antiserum (TAT). As in other species infection with *C. tetani* can follow wounds other than castration wounds, but in pigs this is extremely rare.

Pigs will show some slight stiffness in gait and have a straight tail and pricked ears. This may progress to recumbency and opisthotonos with all the limbs rigid and pointing backwards. As death normally follows, euthanasia must be advised. However, in many cases recumbency does not occur and the pigs with or without treatment with penicillin and TAT will recover.

Clostridium novyi type B will affect pigs and cause sudden death in adults and large fattening pigs. *C. novyi* type A may also cause similar deaths. Both organisms seem to produce very powerful toxins after multiplication in the pig's liver. This is thought to occur if the liver does not receive sufficient oxygen as a result of chronic pneumonia. *C. novyi* infection may also follow any enteritis caused by another organism. Diagnosis can be made on post-mortem. The carcass will show rapid putrefaction with submandibular swelling, pulmonary oedema and an excess of pericardial and peritoneal fluid, which is often blood tinged. The pathognomonic sign is the famous 'Aero liver'. FAT or PCR techniques can be used to confirm the diagnosis.

Clostridium septicum has been isolated from pigs which have shown gangrenous swelling of the limbs. These cases are normally fatal and euthanasia is advised.

Pigs will contract botulism but it is extremely rare. *Clostridium botulinum* multiplies and produces its toxin anaerobically in organic matter outside the pig. The pig is contaminated with toxin by ingesting it in the food. Affected pigs normally show the main sign which is flaccid paralysis within 24 h of ingestion of the contaminated food. Initially this paralysis will be seen in the front legs and jaws. There will be excessive salivation.

The paralysis will spread to the hind legs and excessive urination will be seen. The anus will be flaccid. If the pig becomes laterally recumbent it should be destroyed as recovery is rarely achieved. However, if the pig has only ingested enough toxin for it to remain in sternal recumbency, with good nursing recovery is possible. Rarely is the antitoxin available for treatment. Antibiotics are not appropriate. Pigs should not be killed for human consumption as the meat will cause botulism in humans. In some countries there is a botulism vaccine available. This can be used on pigs which scavenge on rubbish dumps. This will protect the pigs and their owners who may be tempted to eat affected animals.

Escherichia coli diarrhoea

This is a disease of the neonatal piglet. It normally starts with diarrhoea but quickly progresses to a septicaemia and death if there is no treatment. *Escherichia coli* will cause disease conditions in older pre- and post-weaned piglets. These will be described separately. In the neonatal piglet there are certain specific strains of *E. coli* involved, particularly those with the 'O', 'K', 'H' and 'F' antigens. The disease is often called colisepticaemia. It is the most common cause of enteritis in the pig not only in the UK but also worldwide. The bacteria are found in the intestines of normal healthy adult animals. They will infect the small intestine of the non-immune piglet and produce a toxin. The piglet will have diarrhoea and will rapidly become very ill. This may occur within a few hours of birth. They may die so quickly with convulsions that the clinician may be misled and consider neurological conditions or poisoning. Post-mortem may reveal meningitis. *E. coli* will be able to be grown in pure culture from heart blood, liver and spleen. Laboratory confirmation is important for the strain, so that the appropriate vaccine can be given to the sow, and the sensitivity, so that the appropriate antibiotic can be given to the piglets.

The disease may not be peracute but just acute with watery diarrhoea. The piglets will be visibly dehydrated but may continue to suck. Death will occur in 48 h. However some may recover and regain condition. Electrolytes as well as antibiotics are vital for treatment. The outbreak will continue until the sows and gilts coming to the farrowing quarters have been vaccinated. There will be lateral spread from neighbouring litters. The infection will follow inadequately cleaned farrowing pens. Post-mortem will reveal a dehydrated piglet with milk in its stomach. Infarctions in the wall of the stomach are not pathognomonic but very suggestive of *E. coli* infection. A definitive diagnosis cannot be made without ruling out other organisms, e.g. viruses and protozoa.

Treatment with oral antibiotics, namely spectromycin, neomycin or enrofloxacin, which are prepared in a special pump form, may be adequate or may have to be supplemented by a parenteral injection initially.

Control should be based on good hygiene and an 'all-in all-out' system in the whole farrowing shed. Although the condition is not nearly so common in outdoor pigs, a strict 'turn and burn' should be used with the farrowing huts. There are a wide variety of vaccines available which need to be given to the pregnant sow to provide passive immunity in the colostrum. It is vital that the vaccine contains the correct antigens for the outbreak in question. Practitioners should work closely with the laboratory.

E. coli may cause diarrhoea any time up until weaning. The faeces are often grey or white and hence the name 'white scour'. The disease is much more common in piglets fed replacement diets. It may also occur if the temperature in the creep area of the farrowing house is too cold. In these cases often the pigs do not receive sufficient colostrum. Piglets will also not receive sufficient colostrum if the sow is ill with farrowing fever. The disease in this older age group of piglets does not normally have a high mortality, although haemorrhagic diarrhoea will occur and wipe out whole litters. Once again practitioners should make sure there is no other organism which is infecting the piglets. Other organisms may be more important than the *E. coli*. Vaccination may still have a role in prevention in this disease. Electrolytes are again useful, as is antibiotic medicated feed.

E. coli may affect pigs in the post-weaning period but in the author's experience it very rarely has a high mortality. It nearly always occurs after mixing batches of pigs after weaning. Diagnosis relies on growing pure growths of β-haemolytic strains. These are not actually easy to grow from the faeces. They are only grown from the gut contents of a pig at post-mortem. They will not be found in any other organs. Prompt treatment is important to avoid growth checks. Antibiotics should be given in the water rather than the food, as often the pigs are anorexic to some degree and therefore will not ingest a sufficient quantity of the antibiotic in the food. However, they are always thirsty.

Sow vaccination in post-weaning infections is not helpful. Rigid attention to detail to the environment of newly weaned pigs is vital. They should be warm and not subjected to draughts. Groups should be mixed as little as possible. The creep feed should initially be the same in the post-weaning period as the creep fed while the piglets were with the sow. All changes to the feed should be made very gradually. Various oral non-antibiotic preparations are suggested for prevention, e.g. probiotics and zinc oxide. Antimicrobial growth promoters are banned in the EU but are licensed elsewhere. Only experimental vaccines are available at the present time. However it is hoped that one will soon be available.

The final *E. coli* enteric disease to be seen in pigs is oedema disease often called bowel oedema. It is a condition seen in very rapidly growing newly weaned pigs. It is caused by *E. coli* strains which produce verotoxin. This toxin is taken up by the walls of the arteries and weakens them, allowing fluid to leave the circulation and cause oedema of the tissues. The eyelids will be oedematous and the squeak will be higher pitched. As there will be oedema in the brain, the condition may be seen as a neurological condition.

The condition normally occurs within a week of weaning and affects the best pigs in the group. Pigs may be found dead. Careful examination will reveal the peripheral oedema and dullness followed by head pressing and blindness. The pigs will then go into lateral recumbency and have paddling leg movement before death. Normally the rectal temperature is not raised. Diarrhoea is not a feature.

The oedema will be seen clearly on post-mortem. This is pathognomonic if seen in the stomach wall, the larynx and the kidney capsule. The oedema can be confirmed histologically. Diagnosis can be endorsed by growth of the appropriate strains of *E. coli* from the small intestine.

Once pigs show neurological signs, there is little hope of recovery. Antibiotics such as amoxicillin will help, if given promptly prior to neurological signs. The remaining pigs should be given a less nutritious diet.

Helicobacter infection

Helicobacter spp., namely *H. heilmannii* and *H. pametensis*, have been isolated from pigs. Their significance is not known but it is likely that they will cause some gastritis. Ulcers in the stomach have not been found. Experimentally pigs can be infected with the human pathogen *Helicobacter pylori*. It has never been isolated from pigs in natural circumstances but in theory *Helicobacter* spp. from pigs could infect humans.

Proliferative enteropathy

Proliferative enteropathy (PE) is not a simple condition. It is an infectious bacterial condition of the mucosa of the small and large bowel. It underlies necrotic enteritis, regional ileitis and proliferative haemorrhagic enteropathy (PHE). It occurs worldwide. There is a high incidence in herds in many countries, both in studies made on herds but also in studies made at abattoirs. There is evidence that 90–100% of pig farms in the UK are infected with the organism. It may well be a stress-related syndrome. The causal bacterium, *Lawsonia intracellularis*, as the name suggests, is intracellular. It may well live under the right conditions outside cells but it can only multiply when it is intracellular. It is an enteric organism and infection occurs *per os* (po). The incubation period can be as short as 4 days but normally it is considerably longer. The organism is not shed until 2 weeks after infection. There is mucosal proliferation causing erosions in the ileum. The muscular coats become hyperplastic, giving the classic appearance of 'hosepipe gut'. Recently weaned pigs are the most commonly affected age group. Affected pigs lose weight and appear pale, and yet they do not lose their appetite. They may well vomit. They will be anaemic as a result of the melaena which is easily recognized by the blackened faeces. They may die suddenly with clotted blood in the small bowel. Those that do not die may be always stunted and so euthanasia is advised. The majority will recover in a month. When the disease enters the breeding herd for the first time there may be abortions.

When pigs die the diagnosis of PE can be made from the main post-mortem finding of the thickened flaccid ileum and proximal spiral colon. The mucosa will have the classic thickening. However clinicians have to go further and suggest whether the lining of the intestine is covered with yellow or grey friable masses, indicating necrotic enteritis; whether the wall of the ileum is smooth, i.e. hosepipe gut indicating regional ileitis; or whether the ileum is distended with clotted blood, indicating PHE. The clinician can take histopathological sections to confirm the visual diagnosis. In the live animal the presence of the disease can be confirmed by PCR on the faeces.

The disease is spread from herd to herd by carrier animals. It is just possible that vectors might be involved, as rodents can be infected experimentally.

Treatment of the individual pig is best carried out with long-acting tetracycline by intramuscular injection. Tetracyclines or tylosin are the antibiotics of choice for group therapy in the drinking water. Some authorities favour tiamulin or lincomycin, particularly if there are other enteric pathogens involved. Tetracyclines may be effective given in the feed but levels should be higher than standard, in the region of 600 ppm for a minimum of 2 weeks.

The best method of control is using oral vaccination. Antibiotic growth promoters e.g. virginamycin are used to good effect in countries outside the EU, but the author is not in favour of this approach.

Salmonellosis

This is a real problem in pigs, particularly in the UK. The isolation rate from abattoir surveys indicates that the UK has one of the highest rates in the EU. Quoting rates is not worthwhile as they can alter radically in a very short time span. Also on mainland Europe, pigs are often reared and fattened in one country but slaughtered in a different country. The figures will then not be accurate.

The nomenclature of *Salmonella* spp. found in pigs is not straightforward. The specific pig salmonella used to be called *Salmonella choleraesuis*. Pig salmonella are now all called *Salmonella enterica* with different serotypes. So *S. choleraesuis* is now called *S. enterica* serovar Choleraesuis. There are several other important serovars, namely Typhimurium, Derby, Arizona, Heidelberg and Typhisuis. There are also others. The various serovars vary in importance in each country. The serovars are classified on their somatic antigens ('O' antigens) and their flagella antigens ('H' antigens). Salmonella can be differentiated even further by their phage type.

Salmonellosis can be classified into three clinical types: (i) enteritis which is either caused by or will cause a septicaemia; (ii) enteritis which will involve local invasion outside the intestine; and (iii) a subclinical type where the salmonella just multiply in the intestine but do not cause enteritis. It should not be forgotten that salmonella can gain entry via the respiratory route.

The serovars which cause the most serious and rapid destruction of mucosal cells, e.g. Typhimurium, are more likely to cause the most serious enteritis. The septicaemic form is much more common in younger pigs relatively soon after weaning, i.e. in the 10- to 16-week-old range. They may be found dead. This form certainly causes a high morbidity and mortality. There is a high fever sometimes with pneumonic signs as well as diarrhoea. There may also be neurological signs and severe skin discoloration. Recovered pigs will be weak and severely emaciated. Their extremities, e.g. tails and ears, which have been discoloured, will slough off. The diarrhoea will persist and the pigs will huddle under the straw for warmth.

Cases of less acute salmonellosis do not cause septicaemia. Diarrhoea is, however, always a feature. Cases will occur in a wide variety of age ranges even in unweaned piglets. The diarrhoea is normally creamy. Dysentery is rarely seen but some necrotic sloughing of the mucosa may occur. Some clinicians maintain that pigs suffering from this less acute salmonellosis have a distinct smell but this has not been the author's experience. Rectal stricture is often reported in the literature but the author has never observed this. Naturally in these cases euthanasia must be advised.

Post-mortem findings reflect the severity of the disease. In the septicaemic form where sudden death has occurred, the pigs are in good condition. There are often colour changes in the ears. There will be multiple haemorrhages seen throughout the carcass. The mesenteric lymph nodes will be swollen and haemorrhagic. There will be splenic enlargement and sub-peritoneal haemorrhages on the surface of the spleen. The focal necrotic changes often suggested by other authors have not been seen by the author except when histopathological samples have been sent to the laboratory. In the less acute disease the small intestine will be inflamed and contain very watery contents. Often there is gastric ulceration. Petechiae are often seen on the liver and kidneys. Both of these organs are often pale. In the more chronic form the almost pathognomonic sign is button ulcers at the ileo-caecal junction. In the almost subclinical form the only changes which will be seen will be inflammation of the small intestine and some swelling of the mesenteric lymph nodes.

Laboratory confirmation is important in this zoonotic disease. Any salmonella isolate is significant from a zoonotic standpoint. However for a proper diagnosis salmonella organisms need to be isolated from any part of the carcass outside the intestines. Large numbers of salmonella need to be cultured from the intestinal contents or from the faeces for a confirmed diagnosis to be made. It should be remembered that pigs in many herds do not show disease signs. The ELISA test using 'O' antigens can be used on serum or meat juice and is a useful screening test.

Sick animals can be treated with many types of antibiotic injections on a daily basis. This can be followed up with water medication. However every effort should be made to grow the specific salmonella and test for resistance. Then the correct antibiotic can be given in adequate doses to avoid the build-up of antibiotic-resistant bacteria. Practitioners in the UK should remember that nitrofurazone, furazolidone and chloramphenicol may not be used.

Hygiene precautions are very important. Practitioners should prepare a specific salmonella herd control plan. This should be updated on a regular basis taking into account the clinical disease on the farm, the ELISA results from the slaughtered pigs and any new stock coming on to the farm. Total depopulation with repopulation with salmonella-free stock is unlikely to be a realistic option. However careful attention to detail suggested in the herd health plan can bring encouraging results.

Swine dysentery

This is a condition of larger growing pigs and adults. It is caused by *Brachyspira* (used to be called *Sepulina* or *Treponema*) *hyodysenteriae*. As the name suggests, dysentery is a feature. Mucus is also passed, often containing some necrotic material.

It occurs worldwide. The organism requires moisture to survive outside the body. It is easily carried on dirty wellington boots. Infection occurs orally. The target organ is the colon. The organism multiplies in the mucosal crypts and causes inflammation and loss of tissue, allowing blood to seep into the lumen of the large bowel. The incubation period can be as short as a week but may be up to 8 weeks. The infected pigs will show a high fever and quickly die without treatment. Initially there is diarrhoea which quickly turns to dysentery. Infected pigs appear gaunt with sunken eyes and flanks. Mainly the pigs are anorexic but they are always thirsty. Wet fed pigs will start urine drinking which makes the condition much worse. Survivors may be permanently stunted and have intermittent diarrhoea. They can remain as carriers for several months. It is mainly a disease of fat pigs but it may affect naive sows, particularly near to parturition or in early lactation. On post-mortem the pigs will be in poor condition. The large bowel will be swollen and full of liquid faeces and blood. The mucosa will be diphtheritic and the serosal surface will be dark purple and oedematous. The mesenteric lymph nodes will be swollen and pale. The organisms can be seen in wet smears taken from freshly dead animals. They can be seen on histopathological samples stained with special stains. Diagnosis in live animals can be confirmed on wet smears taken from fresh faeces. Culture requires special bacteriological techniques. ELISA tests are available for herd screening.

Tylosin used to be the drug of choice for treatment either of the individual by injection or for the group in the water. Sadly most isolates are now resistant to tylosin, so tiamulin either as an injection or in the water would now be the drug of choice.

Control in the short term can be carried out with tiamulin or valnemulin in the feed. However what is really required is a radical improvement in the general hygiene with the use of an 'all-in all-out' system. There are no vaccines available. Depopulation and restocking is a possibility. This may not be required with the use of a medicated early weaning system.

Spirochaetal diarrhoea

It is difficult to separate this condition from swine dysentery. By definition it is caused by spirochetes other than *B. hyodysenteriae*. In this disease dysentery is nothing like so marked. There is often no fever and deaths are rare. The disease is found throughout the world. The two main pathogens are *Brachyspira intermedia* and *Brachyspira pilosicoli*. Whereas *B. hyodysenteriae* is strongly β-haemolytic, these two organisms are only weakly β-haemolytic. The disease is really very similar to swine dysentery. Infection is via the oral route but the inflammation in the large bowel is only mild. *Trichuris suis* infection seems to potentiate the disease which is normally seen in young newly weaned pigs. It has an incubation period of 1 to 3 weeks. Pigs will be off food and have a tucked-up appearance. There is normally a low fever. Morbidity is high but mortality is less than 1% and recovery occurs within a week. Post-mortems are unrewarding with just some oedema of the large bowel. The organisms may be found on histopathological sections of the large bowel using special stains. *B. intermedia* and *B. pilosicoli* can survive better in the natural environment than *B. hyodysenteriae* and therefore biosecurity is even more important. It is possible that *B. intermedia* and *B. pilosicoli* are zoonotic. However, it may be that there are different strains in humans. Certainly the organisms have been found in rodents and so rodent control is important. Practitioners should stress to pig keepers the need to wash their hands before eating and drinking.

Diagnosis is best performed clinically with laboratory support. It is important from a long-term point of view to separate spirochaetal diarrhoea from swine dysentery. Once again there is no vaccine available and treatment is the same as for swine dysentery.

Yersinia infection

This can cause human disease and in very rare cases can cause disease in pigs. The two main organisms are *Yersinia enterocolitica* and *Yersinia pseudotuberculosis*. The organisms are very commonly found in normal pigs at slaughter throughout the world. They have been associated with mild diarrhoea in pigs. The large bowel is affected. In very rare cases there is a septicaemia with small abscesses in the liver and mesenteric lymph nodes. There will be a slightly raised rectal temperature with blood-stained diarrhoea. Diagnosis will be on isolation of the organism but interpretation needs to be given with care as the organism is commonly found in normal pigs. It is only significant if found in large numbers and linked with clinical signs. Pigs even with septicaemia will self-cure. Antibiotics and supportive treatment are rarely required. The organism affects rodents so their control is important. Human hygiene is important. The preparation of an autogenous vaccine has been reported.

Enteric Diseases Caused by Protozoa

Coccidiosis

This occurs in baby pigs. There are eight *Eimeria* and one *Isospora* species affecting pigs, but only *Isospora suis* is considered to be of clinical importance. It is the most common parasitic cause of neonatal diarrhoea worldwide. Upon ingestion of infective oocysts, the parasite invades the epithelium of the small intestine. It is an obligatory intracellular protozoan. The parasite multiplies rapidly to form more oocysts which sporulate in the environment to become infective. It has a prepatent period of less than 1 week. Infections can occur in the first days of life. It then causes profuse non-haemorrhagic diarrhoea. The most common time for the infection is in 7- to 10-day-old unweaned piglets. Weight gains are depressed. Although the infection is self-limiting, unthrifty piglets and uneven litter weights will cause considerable economic loss and will be a welfare issue. Coccidiosis occurs only in the first 3 weeks of life; however the damage to the intestine may well cause problems for a much longer period of time. There is a distinct age-related resistance to the disease due to a primary immune response to *I. suis*. This seems to be dependent on T cells which are found in the mucosa of the gut of infected piglets in large numbers. There is a subsequent development of cellular immunological memory. There are two licensed products: (i) toltrazuril, which can be given as one-off oral dose of 20 mg/kg at 3–5 days of age; and (ii) sulfadiazine/trimethropin, which can be given as a single intramuscular injection of 25 mg sulfadiazine and 5 mg trimethropin per 2 kg. Improving the hygiene of the farrowing accommodation will help reduce the incidence of the condition.

Treatment significantly improves piglet health and weight gain. However, treating the sows is not helpful. It is hoped that a vaccine will be developed to control this disease as an alternative treatment.

Cryptosporidiosis

This is caused by *Cryptosporidium parvum*. The organism is present in healthy pigs but has been found in large numbers in piglets with diarrhoea. It is found throughout the world. Infection is via the oral route. Healthy pigs will harbour the organism. It is seen in 2- to 3-week-old pigs. They will be depressed and pass watery diarrhoea. They do not have raised rectal temperatures. The organism can be seen on faecal smears using specific stains. Post-mortems are unremarkable except for some inflammation of the small intestine. The organism may be seen on histopathological sections of the small bowel. The organism is very resistant and will remain in slurry for many months. Good farrowing accommodation hygiene is important and may well be all that is required for control. There are no licensed medicines in the UK but halofuginone lactate can be given orally under the cascade principle at 1 mg/10 kg. It should be remembered that this is a zoonotic disease.

Enteric Diseases Caused by Endoparasites

Ascariasis

This is caused by this large roundworm *Ascaris suum*, which is extremely common throughout the world. It actually only rarely causes ill thrift in growing pigs but does cause liver condemnation at slaughter.

The worms can be as long as 40 cm. Their eggs are extremely resistant to the environment and can live for many years away from the pig, so eradication is unlikely to be successful. The worm has a direct life cycle. After the eggs are ingested by the pig, the larvae emerge and migrate into the mucosa of the caecum within a few hours.

They then rapidly migrate to the liver where they moult and proceed to the lungs. They become fourth-stage larvae within the large airways of the lungs. They are then coughed up and swallowed to become adult worms in the small intestine. Normally the coughing is transitory. However it may alarm pet pig owners or smallholders, who may mistake the condition for respiratory disease. The prepatent period is 50 days. Clinically mature worms in the bowel do not normally cause any clinical signs. The mature worms will be seen on post-mortem as adults in the small intestine. In extremely rare cases large numbers may cause an obstruction of the small intestine resulting in death. Also in rare cases the worms will be seen to block the bile ducts causing jaundice. The small white fibrotic lesions seen in the liver, called 'milk spots', will take 6 weeks to dissolve after the larvae have passed through the liver. They do not affect the pig but cause condemnations at the abattoir. Transmission is normally from weaner to weaner rather than sow to offspring. Confirmation of the disease is by high faecal worm egg counts (FECs). There is an ELISA test available.

As stated earlier, ascarid eggs are extremely resistant and can survive on fields for many years. In buildings pressure-washing without thorough drying enhances survival of eggs. Flaming on concrete is a good method of control.

Treatment can be either by injection or orally in the water or the feed. Ivermectins may be given im at 300 µg/kg and doramectin can be given im at 0.3 mg/kg. Flubendazole can be given in the water at 1 mg/kg for 5 days. Practitioners should liaise with food suppliers for in-feed medication. Adults should be treated every 6 months. Treatment during lactation or pregnancy does not cause problems. Weaners and fatteners should be treated every 2 months, with careful attention to withhold times for slaughter.

Hyostronylosis

This disease is caused by *Hyostrongylus rubidus*, the red stomach worm, and mainly affects adults. The worms are 1 cm in length and may cause gastric ulceration and ill thrift. The worm has a direct life cycle with typical strongyle eggs which develop on the ground. When eaten further development occurs in the gastric mucosal glands. The prepatent period is 2 weeks. Heavily infected sows will suffer severe weight loss. They will show high FECs. This occurs particularly in lactating sows. Some authorities consider there is a hormone influence on the larval development. Severe infections may actually cause anaemia and anorexic sows. These animals will be very white and have black faeces. They do not have loose motions but may have depraved appetites. On post-mortem the stomach will contain large numbers of worms and the gastric mucosa will be pitted. This has classically been described as a 'Morocco leather' appearance. Although this worm will occur in housed sows it is really a parasite of outdoor sows.

Treatment can be either by injection or orally in the water or the feed. Ivermectins may be given im at 300 µg/kg and doramectin can be given im at 0.3 mg/kg. Flubendazole can be given in the water at 1 mg/kg for 5 days. Practitioners should liaise with food suppliers for in-feed medication.

As the parasite is a problem in outdoor sows, it is suggested that they are wormed in June and December. Weaners need not be wormed. If practitioners are in any doubt about infections FECs should be performed.

Oesophagostomosis

The worms *Oesophagostomum dentatum* and *Oesophagostomum quadrispinulatum* cause this disease. They are the nodular worms which mainly live in the colon and caecum of adult pigs. They occur throughout the world, particularly in pigs kept in poor conditions both indoors and outdoors. The worms are about 1.5 cm in length, may cause ill thrift and have been cited as a cause of torsion of the colon. They have a direct life cycle. The prepatent period is 3 weeks. They are a problem in sows. Heavy worm burdens are rare but will cause diarrhoea. They may cause loss of weight and loss of milk. They do not normally cause a problem in weaners or fatteners. They may cause high FECs. On post-mortem they will be seen in the large intestine. Classically they form nodules in the mucosa. The infective larvae do not survive for long in the environment particularly on dry concrete. Indoors, however, larval development will occur all through the year. Outdoors, larval development is restricted to the summer and autumn.

This disease shows an epidemiological phenomenon of a 'periparturient rise'. As parturition approaches the sows will show much greater worm egg output. Therefore treatment ideally should be carried out just before farrowing. Treatment can be by injection or orally in the water or the feed. Ivermectins may be given im at 300 μg/kg and doramectin can be given im at 0.3 mg/kg. Flubendazole can be given in the water at 1 mg/kg for 5 days. Practitioners should liaise with food suppliers for in-feed medication. These worms may be spread by rats and by wild boar.

Trichuris suis infestation

This is the pig whipworm, which is about 1.5 cm long and lives in the caecum. It only causes problems in young growing pigs if there are heavy infestations. The worm is found worldwide. It will cause diarrhoea and poor weight gains. It is normally only a problem with poor management. The gut may become ulcerated and high FECs will be seen. Infection is via the oral route. The adult worm lives in the large bowel. Eggs are eaten and reach the large bowel where there are several larval stages. The prepatent period is 6 to 8 weeks. Clinical signs are rare and are normally as a result of another enteric organism. Adult worms will be seen in the large intestine. The females are larger and are up to 8 cm long. The mucosa may be inflamed. Diagnosis can be by FECs being raised. There is a specific ELISA. The worm affects indoor and outdoor pigs as well as wild boar. It should not be forgotten that it is a zoonotic worm. Human infection is rare.

Treatment can be either by injection or orally in the water or the feed. Ivermectins may be given im at 300 μg/kg and doramectin can be given im at 0.3 mg/kg. Flubendazole can be given in the water at 1 mg/kg for 5 days. Practitioners should liaise with food suppliers for in-feed medication.

Resistance and control

So far, resistance of helminths to anthelmintics has not been found as a problem in pigs. Treatment should be carried out in adults on a 6-monthly basis, with outdoor pigs being moved to clean pasture and indoor pigs having their accommodation steam-cleaned and very importantly dried, ideally with a flame gun. Growing pigs should be treated at 8 weeks of age and then every 2 months until maturity. As with all medication meat withdrawal periods must be followed, so that timing of anthelmintic treatments may be critical. All treatments must be recorded in the medicine book.

It is important to remember to reduce the risk of resistance by treating animals up to weight. Therefore when treating individuals or pens of pigs the dosage of the anthelmintic should be worked out for the heaviest in the group. Only licensed medicines for pigs should be used.

Control of helminths in pigs can be easily accomplished in commercial herds by in-feed ivermectin or fenbendazole given at 6-monthly intervals.

Individual treatments can be given by im injection of doramectin at 0.3 mg/kg or by sc injection of ivermectin at 300 μg/kg.

Small group treatment may be carried out with in-water medication of flubendazole at 1 mg/kg for 5 days or fenbendazole oral pellets at 5 mg/kg as a single dose.

Enteric Diseases of Unknown Aetiology

Bowel torsion

This is a condition of adults or larger fat pigs. They are normally found dead or *in extremis*. They will be in lateral recumbency, tachycardic and with acute dyspnoea.

Rectal temperature will be very subnormal. Treatment is hopeless and euthanasia should be carried out without delay. The most common torsion is the whole of the spiral colon on its axis. Pigs will also sustain small bowel torsion. Gastric torsion is rare but is normally seen only on post-mortem. Splenic torsion may also be seen.

Colitis

This syndrome occurs in growing pigs and is normally related to a change of diet. It is particularly linked with pellet-based diets rather than meal diets. The main clinical sign is soft faeces with intermittent diarrhoea. The pigs will be tucked up and obviously off colour. The faeces may be extra slimy or frothy. On post-mortem it is not only the colon which is affected but also the small intestine. The contents will be bubbly and oily. Histopathology is unrewarding. Many enteric pathogens have been implicated but none is consistent. Antibiotics and NSAIDs do not seem to help the disease. Dexamethazone gives a temporary improvement. The main method of control is either to change to a meal if pelleted feed is being fed or to return the pigs to their previous ration. Often the condition will disappear on its own.

Gastric torsion

This is a disease of sows and is linked to once daily feeding. Sows are often found dead or *in extremis*. They appear bloated. There is often evidence of acute pain but normally this is missed by the pig keeper. The aetiology is not known but rapid fermentation of large volumes of food is likely to be the cause. Several deaths may be recorded. On post-mortem the stomach will be very distended and haemorrhagic. Torsion is often actually not seen. Sometimes there is torsion of the spleen. There is no useful treatment although if there is no torsion forced exercise and liquid paraffin may be tried. The condition can be prevented by twice daily feeding.

Gastric ulcers

These are a common finding in normal pigs at slaughter. Their significance is therefore in doubt. However, there is definitely a clinical entity where a gastric ulcer will perforate and haemorrhage into the lumen, resulting in death or severe disease.

The aetiology of gastric ulcers is very obscure. There is no doubt that certain other serious conditions such as CSF and salmonellosis will cause gastric ulcers, but ulcers will occur when there has been no history of these diseases. Copper used to be added to the diet of pigs and was thought to be a possible cause, but the condition is still just as prevalent today in the UK and copper has not been added to pig diets for some years. High levels of oxidized unsaturated fatty acids in the diet may well play a part in the aetiology of the condition. There is a definite correlation with the use of wheat feeds in its occurrence. The author considers feed particle size, season, stress and starvation not to be likely causes of the disease as from his records there is no evidence to link any of these causes with an increase in the disease.

It is a peracute disease with the majority of animals being found dead or *in extremis*. They have a severely low rectal temperature and completely pale mucous membranes. They are normally in lateral recumbency grinding their teeth. On post-mortem the stomach and small intestine are filled with blood. Perforation into the peritoneum is rare but in these cases the abdomen is filled with blood. The author has seen the condition only in large fat pigs or in adults.

Intestinal haemorrhagic syndrome

This is a condition which is normally associated with the feeding of whey, but it is also seen rarely in pigs fed on other regimens. It is commonly called 'whey bloat' or 'bloody gut'. It is a peracute disease of fattening pigs. They are often found dead. The causal organism might be *C. perfringens* type A. On post-mortem the small intestine is distended with blood-stained fluid. It is often linked with intestinal torsion. Treatment has been recommended with oxytetracycline at 20 mg/kg given im by injection. The author has not found this to be useful even with injections of NSAIDs. Control is to reduce the amount of whey in the diet.

Rectal prolapse

See Chapter 7.

Rectal stricture

This condition, in the author's experience, follows a rectal prolapse. However, some pig keepers claim that certain affected pigs have never suffered a rectal prolapse. Affected pigs become anorexic and dull. They will appear to be bloated. Often they pass a ribbon of faeces. On post-mortem the whole of the large bowel will be full of ingesta. It appears to be a physical problem just like a blocked drain. The condition may be linked with damage to the spine as the author has seen the condition in paraplegic pigs. Confirmation of the condition will be made when taking a rectal temperature and observing the small diameter of the rectum. The author has attempted treatment with primitive surgery using local anaesthetic by inserting a lubricated gloved finger into the rectum and manually dilating the stricture. This treatment is followed up with oral liquid paraffin. Antibiotics and NSAIDs may be helpful.

9 Diseases of the Respiratory and Circulatory Systems

Respiratory Diseases

Introduction

Respiratory disease is extremely prevalent in commercial growing and fattening pigs. It accounts for a considerable amount of deaths and perhaps more importantly of lower growth rates. The importance of respiratory disease is not so high in outdoor pigs and is of little importance in pet pigs. The predominant signs are dyspnoea, tachycardia, pyrexia and coughing (Fig. 9.1). There are other signs which are not seen in all respiratory diseases, e.g. blueing of the ears and twisting of the snout. Signs of respiratory disease will lead to other problems, e.g. violent coughing will lead to rectal prolapse and twisting of the snout will lead to a nasal discharge. Diagnosis on history and clinical signs may be possible but confirmation is likely to require post-mortems coupled with virus and bacterial examination. Respiratory health status of a herd can be made by lung examination of slaughtered pigs at the abattoir or by group blood sampling.

The mode of infection is from pig to pig, i.e. mixing of pigs. This can be at an on-farm level or by incoming pigs. In small herds there is always a danger from pigs going to shows or the borrowing of a boar. Some respiratory disease may be airborne and carried on the wind.

Prevention is best achieved by keeping a closed herd and by carrying out strict biosecurity. Veterinary surgeons should be mindful of not risking the introduction of disease by their routine visit. Ideally they should be 'pig free' for 3 days before a visit to a high health status herd. Vaccination is extremely useful. Good ventilation and temperature control are vital. Antibiotics should be used responsibly. A study in Belgium (Del Pozo Sacristan et al., 2012) demonstrated that chlortetracycline was able to decrease the prevalence of pneumonia lesions when administered in the feed during two alternate weeks starting at the onset of clinical respiratory disease. Performance losses and clinical signs in a herd infected with Mycoplasma hyopneumoniae were numerically, but not significantly, reduced.

The causes of respiratory disease are, in the main, viruses, bacteria and endoparasites.

Respiratory Diseases Caused by Viruses

Inclusion body rhinitis

Inclusion body rhinitis (IBR) is a very rare respiratory disease which is lethal to young piglets but signs, except transitory sneezing, are rarely seen in adults. It is also called porcine cytomegalovirus infection (PCMV). As the name suggests, it is caused by a

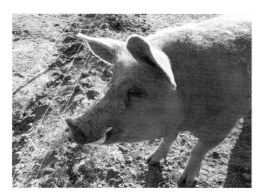

Fig. 9.1. A pig in respiratory distress.

cytomegalovirus. The virus is found worldwide with up to 90% of herds in the UK affected. However, clinical signs are rarely seen. The virus may be spread across the placenta causing early embryonic death. There is sow-to-sow transfer and also boar-to-sow transfer. In naive herds baby pigs under 2 weeks of age will show respiratory signs. These include rhinitis, sneezing and respiratory distress. Up to a quarter of the litter may die. If weaner pigs are infected they will be ill with anorexia, pyrexia, coughing and have a nasal discharge. Virus may be isolated from the nasal discharge, which is often purulent and may sometimes contain blood. Postmortem will reveal a serious rhinitis, but there is no damage to the turbinates or twisting of the snout. The diagnosis can be confirmed by an ELISA or PCR. There is no vaccine available but once a herd has experience an outbreak the clinical signs seem to disappear. Abortion rates are low. Clinicians might advise antibiotics for the secondary infections in the face of an outbreak to lessen the mortality in the baby pigs.

Porcine reproductive and respiratory syndrome

This is a very serious syndrome caused by an arterivirus. It is also called porcine epidemic abortion and respiratory syndrome (PEARS). It is known to pig keepers in the UK as 'blue ear'. As the name implies, PRRS will cause reproductive problems in sows and respiratory signs in fattening pigs. It is found throughout the world except it is not seen in

Australia or New Zealand. The main spread of the infection is by pig-to-pig contact using the respiratory route. It can also be spread venereally and by AI. The adult pigs do not normally show a fever but laboured breathing and inappetence for 2–4 days. The infection will spread through a whole herd of adults in 10 days. There will be early embryonic deaths, abortions and stillbirths. Skin changes occur more commonly in growing pigs, showing the classic blue ear appearance. Baby pigs often show oedema of the eyelids and conjunctivitis. Mortality may not be high in well-managed herds. The post-mortem picture may well be confusing as often there are other respiratory pathogens involved. ELISA and PCR will confirm the diagnosis. Serology retrospectively may be helpful after an abortion storm particularly if rising titres can be demonstrated. Being a viral disease there must be secondary bacterial infection, but treatment with a variety of antibiotics is rarely helpful. NSAIDs certainly have a place for treatment. Injectable preparations may be given to individual bad cases. Treatment with oral paracetamol or aspirin in the early stages is worthwhile. There are several commercial vaccines available, which are very effective.

Post-weaning multisystemic wasting syndrome

Post-weaning multisystemic wasting syndrome (PMWS) is extremely important in commercial pigs. It is caused by a circavirus. It is obviously important in backyard pet pigs obtained from commercial stock. There is a vaccine available. Ideally backyard fattening pigs should be vaccinated before movement. Naturally, good hygiene practices should be paramount, as well as avoiding stress. Once the pigs are showing signs antibiotic treatment is rarely worthwhile and so euthanasia should be carried out. PMWS, as the name suggests, is a multisystemic disease (see Chapter 13).

Swine influenza

These viruses are specific to pigs. They are influenza A viruses. The common strains are

H1N1, H1N2 and H3N2. They causes coughing and dyspnoea. These viruses are found in Europe, Asia and North America. They are not found in Australia or New Zealand. The virus enters the upper respiratory tract and multiplies in the bronchial epithelium. There is a viraemia. Often the disease is made considerably worse by other infections, e.g. viruses like PRRS, bacteria like *Pasteurella multocida* and parasites like ascarids. The virus may damage fetuses *in utero*, causing abortions and stillbirths.

The fever is very severe for the first 24 h with rectal temperatures up to 42°C and many pigs in an outbreak will be prostrate. Coughing may be severe enough to cause vomiting. The conjunctiva will be very inflamed causing excess lacrimation. There may be a bilateral nasal discharge (Fig. 9.2). The disease may blow through in 2 weeks with the majority of the pigs recovering. The few that remain prostrate should be destroyed. In the individual pig warmth will aid recovery which is often quite rapid without treatment. Recovery may be accelerated by injectable or oral NSAIDs including oral aspirin. Adult pigs as well as growing pigs are affected.

On post-mortem severe necrotizing pneumonia will be seen. The virus antigen may be found by reverse transcriptase PCR (RT-PCR). It must be remembered that other pathogens are also likely to be present. The virus may be spread by birds, particularly turkeys. The virus will survive in meat. It should be stressed that meat scraps must not be fed to pigs. There is no licensed vaccine

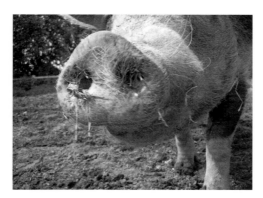

Fig. 9.2. A bilateral nasal discharge.

available in the UK but there are vaccines available in the rest of the world.

Respiratory Diseases Caused by Bacteria

Actinobacillosis

This is a highly contagious respiratory disease, caused by *Actinobacillus pleuropneumoniae*. The disease causes problems worldwide. The bacterium is relatively delicate but will survive outside the body at ambient temperatures in damp conditions. It will also survive in cold fresh water. Transmission is by aerosol or nose-to-nose contact. It is an acute disease with a mortality of 30% in non-immune pigs. There is a fibrinous pleurisy, which may be heard on auscultation. There is a very high rectal temperature. If there is cyanosis death will follow in a few hours. There are often other pathogens involved. If it is not fatal, pigs will show chronic respiratory signs for weeks and will not gain weight, particularly if other respiratory pathogens are involved. Chronically infected pigs should be destroyed on humane grounds.

On post-mortem in acute cases there is a blood-stained fibrinous pleurisy. These lesions become greyish as the disease has developed. Histopathology will show infarcts and alveolar haemorrhages in a bronchopneumonia. Diagnosis can be confirmed on culture. There are several different serotypes which can be separated by ELISA tests. Certain serotypes are more common in different areas, e.g. serotype 2 is the most common serotype found in the UK. Serotypes 8, 3, 6 and 7 are also relatively common.

Antibiotic treatment is rarely effective, as the antibiotics do not reach the affected areas. The organism is actually sensitive to most antibiotics commonly used in pig practice. High doses given for a minimum of 3 days coupled with injectable NSAIDs may help clinical cases. All in-contact pigs must be treated with high doses of the same antibiotic by mouth.

There are commercially available vaccines. Practitioners should be advised to check the serotypes covered by the vaccine against the serotypes which are affecting the pigs.

Atrophic rhinitis

This shows as sneezing in young piglets. It is rarely fatal, but it is progressive and causes atrophy of the turbinate bones with distortion of the nasal septum, resulting in shortening and twisting of the upper jaw. It is caused by a toxigenic strain of *P. multocida*. Deaths occur if there is an additional *Mycoplasma* infection. It is found throughout the world but the incidence is not high. The disease also may be linked with *Bordetella bronchisepitca* infection (see below).

P. multocida is a Gram-negative coccobacillus. Isolation of this organism is not diagnostic per se as it is only certain strains which are toxigenic. The organism is spread by close contact, with the sneezing aiding the spread. Pigs under 2 months of age are affected. The first signs are tear staining and nose bleeds. The twisting of the snout occurs only later in the disease process. The main economical effect of the disease is the poor growth rates. To try to establish the effect of the disease in an infected herd, the snouts of pigs are graded at the abattoir. There are normally five grades of the condition recorded as abnormal. Grade 1 is a slight deviation. Grade 2 is a slight atrophy. Grade 3 is a severe atrophy. Grade 4 is a loss of a turbinate. Grade 5 is a loss of all of the turbinates. When an outbreak is suspected the diagnosis is made mainly on clinical grounds. Practitioners should examine the baby pigs carefully to rule out other causes of damage to the face of the pig. Some of these are congenital, e.g. cleft lip (cheiloschisis), absence of a lower jaw (agnathia) and wry-nose (craniofacial asymmetry). Baby pigs will develop septic conditions in this area due to poor technique used when clipping canine teeth.

A definitive diagnosis can be made from nasal swabs using an ELISA. PCR tests are also available.

Treatment with a variety of antibiotics is effective in reducing the effects of the disease. Oral pumps used over 3 days will be effective, as will single long-acting injections of amoxicillin, enrofloxacin and oxytetracycline. A good control measure is to treat litters of baby pigs with injections of trimethoprim sulfonamide on days 3, 10 and 21. Sows should be vaccinated twice in pregnancy, ideally 5 and 2 weeks before farrowing. Some vaccines are licensed for piglets to be given at 1 and 3 weeks of age.

Bordetella bronchiseptica rhinitis

B. bronchiseptica is an extremely common organism found in the nose of piglets both in the UK and worldwide. It is a Gram-negative aerobic bacillus. It can survive outside the pig for at least 3 weeks in normal conditions. It is spread by direct contact and by aerosol droplets. It affects really young piglets under a week old. It causes sneezing and tear staining. It does not cause physical damage to the snout on its own, only if there is also a toxigenic strain of *P. multocida*. However, lower weight gains are experienced by pigs suffering solely from *B. bronchiseptica*. Older pigs are not affected. No changes are seen on postmortem. Diagnosis is made by culture of the organism from nasal swabs. There are ELISA tests available on serology.

Treatment with most oral antibiotics available in 'pig-pump' form is very effective if continued for 3 days. Vaccination of sows can be carried out with a combined vaccine of a toxigenic strain of *P. multocida* and *B. bronchiseptica*. This killed vaccine should be given in pregnancy at 6 and 2 weeks before parturition. There are live vaccines available for instillation up the nose of day-old piglets but these are not licensed in the UK.

Enzootic pneumonia

This is caused by *M. hyopneumoniae*. It is not only a highly contagious pulmonary disease but also the organism affects the joints. Historically it affected very large numbers of pig herds throughout the world. The clinical incidence has been remarkably reduced by vaccination. The organism can be seen on Giemsa stains. The organism can be detected by pig farmers from nasal swabs (Nathues *et al.*, 2012). It can be spread via aerosols in the wind but it is likely to be seen in pigs soon after arrival on a new holding. They will show mild lameness and/or coughing. Temperatures will be raised initially. Soon the pigs will become normal and stop coughing provided they are in well-ventilated conditions and unless another respiratory pathogen is involved. In these cases they will continue with a respiratory illness which at best will cause reduced weight gains but at worst will cause death or necessitate humane destruction.

Enzootic pneumonia is a herd disease rather than an individual disease. Therefore a diagnosis is normally made as a herd problem. The condition will be seen as continuing pneumonia within a herd. There will be lower than expected growth rates and uneven sizes of pigs within a litter. These signs will be seen in relatively newly weaned pigs. They will be coughing but not actually be ill. There is no pyrexia or dyspnoea. On post-mortem there will be well-demarcated areas of pneumonia in the anterior lobes of the lungs. This will also be seen on routine lung examination at the abattoir. A diagnosis of enzootic pneumonia can be confirmed on culture. It can also be diagnosed on PCR and ELISA. These ELISAs can differentiate *M. hyopneumoniae* from *Mycoplasma flocculare*, *Mycoplasma hyorhinis* and *Mycoplasma hyosynoviae*.

Treatment of enzootic pneumonia is in some ways easy as there are many antibiotics which will treat the disease apparently successfully, but none of them will ever entirely eliminate the organism so that the disease will always return. The use of antibiotics will take time to reduce the lung lesions and restore growth rates but in the end production targets may be met.

There are better methods of control. The well-tried 'all-in all-out' system with treatment on entry will be helpful on a house basis. It will be much more helpful on a whole unit basis. An early weaning system – where the pigs are weaned and moved with treatment to a clean site and reared for 4 weeks, then moved to a grower site for a further 4 weeks before being moved to a clean finisher site – also has merits. Low stocking densities

and outdoor fattening will reduce enzootic pneumonia but both are unlikely to be economic on commercial units.

The ultimate modern method of control is vaccination. There are several commercially available vaccines.

Glasser's disease

This is an infectious disease caused by *Haemophilus parasuis*, which is often fatal in growing pigs. The disease is found throughout the world. It is caused by a Gram-negative coccobacillus. It is non-haemolytic and is hard to culture on blood agar. The agar has to be streaked with a *Staphylococcus* spp. first and then the *H. parasuis* will grow on the edge of the streak as very small clear colonies. The main clinical signs are related to the polyserositis, polyarthritis and sometimes meningitis which can be caused by the organism. The organism also causes an exudative peritonitis and pleurisy. The lung involvement may be shown as bronchitis in adults. The classic scenario is the stressed pig arriving in a contaminated environment. There is a sudden-onset high fever. Lung sounds and pericardial rubbing will be heard on auscultation. Very soon the arthritic signs will be seen. If the pig survives, the disease will be manifest in the joints as a chronic arthritis. Meningitis can occur at this stage. Euthanasia is then the correct procedure. Euthanasia would also be appropriate if there is bowel obstruction from intestinal adhesions. It is a sporadic disease when it occurs on its own, but when animals also have enzootic pneumonia it appears to cause an outbreak with a relatively high morbidity and mortality.

There is a commercially available vaccine either on its own or linked with enzootic pneumonia vaccine.

Mycoplasma hyorhinis disease

This is mainly a disease of young pigs' joints. It does also cause respiratory disease similar to enzootic pneumonia (see above). The organism is found worldwide. It is harder to culture than *M. hyopneumoniae* and therefore may well be missed as it is often present in mixed infection. It enters the pig by the respiratory route and then becomes septicaemic and spreads to the joints and the lungs.

The incubation period is a week. Pigs up to 3 months old will become infected. They will have some pyrexia and general malaise. There is swelling of the joints and lameness. On post-mortem there is often pericarditis, pleurisy and peritonitis as well as inflamed joints. A diagnosis can be made from culture or immunofluorescence of frozen sections of affected lung.

Treatment is the same as for enzootic pneumonia, with oxytetracyclines, tiamulin and tylosine being most commonly used. In the author's experience the injectable route is more effective, particularly if NSAIDs are also injected.

Mycoplasma hyosynoviae disease

This is a disease of older growing pigs between 2 and 5 months of age. It is also mainly a disease of the joints but will cause respiratory signs. It occurs worldwide. It occurs mainly after stress. The organism can be regularly cultured from the tonsil of healthy pigs. There may be coughing and various levels of lameness. One or more joints will be swollen. The organism can be cultured from a joint tap in the live pig or at post-mortem. The lungs may show areas of consolidation. Treatment with injections of tiamulin or tylosin followed by water medication will be helpful. In severe cases NSAIDs are indicated.

Pasteurellosis

This is an infectious disease seen in the older growing pig. It is often secondary to *H. parasuis*, *A. pleuropneumoniae* and *M. hyopneumoniae*. The causal organism is *P. multocida*. However, this can be a primary pathogen not only causing respiratory disease but also septicaemia. This latter manifestation is seen mainly in newly weaned pigs. It may even cause sudden death. In respiratory pasteurellosis there is fever and a nasal discharge. The lung sounds are loud and breathing laboured, often with mouth breathing. Post-mortem will reveal an acute necrotizing and fibrinous pneumonia. Grey areas of consolidation will be seen in the anterior lobes of the lungs. Culture is important not only for diagnosis but also for typing the organism for sensitivity testing. Aggressive antibiotic treatment should be tried using injections of penicillin/ streptomycin or oxytetracycline. Obviously treatment can be changed if there is a sensitivity test result. If there is no sensitivity result available and if treatment is not effective, another antibiotic should be tried. Only when there is improvement seen should injections be stopped and the treatment carried on in the water. In the septicaemic form long-acting antibiotic preparations can be used in the other pigs to try to prevent the condition. There is no vaccine available. Segregated early weaning can be a very effective control method.

Respiratory Diseases Caused by Endoparasites

Ascaris migration

Ascaris suum is not a respiratory endoparasite but its migration phase through the lungs can cause respiratory distress and the parasite is very important in backyard pigs. The signs are similar to asthma in man, heaves in horses or fog fever in cattle, but the pathological lesions are different. With ascaris migration there are just fibrous tracts but no alveolar pathology. Prevention with good helminth control is important and affected pigs should be treated with endoparasiticides.

Metastrongylosis

This disease caused by *Metastrongylus* lungworm is found in outdoor pigs. It rarely causes any respiratory signs or has any effect on growth rates. It is rare as the lungworms are easily controlled by endoparasiticides.

Miscellaneous Causes of Respiratory Disease

Drowning

Pigs can swim but obviously will drown if they become exhausted. It is a myth that they damage their throats with their front hooves. After removal from the water exhausted pigs should be warmed if they are cold. Antibiotics should be given to reduce the risk of inhalation pneumonia. NSAIDs may also aid recovery. Diagnosis can be confirmed on post-mortem by cutting a piece of lung and observing if it will float in water. Normal lung floats. Lung from a drowned pig will sink.

Smoke inhalation

Fires are a constant danger on pig farms, particularly on smallholdings and in old, poorly designed buildings. Pigs will die from smoke inhalation. The cause of death can be seen on post-mortem and confirmed by histopathology. If pigs can be removed from the smoke and are still breathing, they should be given dexamethazone at a raised dose of 1 mg/5 kg. They should be checked to ascertain the extent of any injury from burns. If the percentage of skin damage is >20% they should be destroyed. If not they should be nursed and given antibiotics.

Suffocation

This is a rare cause of death in pigs. The skin in white pigs will be cyanotic. In black pigs, practitioners should examine the mucous membranes. If the pig is still breathing it should be moved to an airy location. There is no other specific treatment.

Diseases of the Circulatory System

Introduction

These diseases are relatively rare in pigs, although pigs are liable to get heart failure when stressed. Hereditary heart diseases are rare.

Autoimmune thrombocytopaenia

This is often called thrombocytopaenic purpura. It is a disease of the newborn after it has ingested the colostrum. It has a very low incidence and is caused by formation by the piglet of antibodies to the antigens produced by the sow. Usually whole litters will die any time within the first week of life. However some smaller piglets may survive if they have not managed to drink some of the colostrum. The piglets will be found dead or *in extremis* with purple patches on the skin and bloody diarrhoea. The mucous membranes will be white and the rectal temperature subnormal.

On post-mortem there are haemorrhages in the lymph nodes, epicardium, myocardium and skeletal muscles, as well as on the skin.

The condition can occur only in litters from sows which have previously had litters from that boar. The condition has been seen only in Large White or Landrace pigs. A definitive diagnosis can be made by a blood test showing reduced platelet counts.

If piglets do look as if they might survive then careful nursing is worthwhile. Although the use of vitamin K has been suggested, in the author's experience it is not useful.

Prevention relies on not mating sows with affected litters to certain boars.

Carbon monoxide poisoning

This occurs mainly when pigs are kept in garages. Pregnant sows are liable to abort. It can occur in baby pigs if gas heaters are faulty. Carbon monoxide affects humans, so care must be taken when dealing with a problem. Turning off the appliance and good ventilation are vital.

- CO > 120 ppm in the air (normal = 50 ppm) causes abortion and an increase in the number of stillbirths.

- CO > 150 ppm causes fetal death as the fetus becomes anoxic. Post-mortems will reveal cherry-red tissues and blood-stained pleural fluids. There is extramedullary haematopoiesis.
- CO > 200 ppm will affect piglets causing lethargy and reduction in growth (Jackson and Cockcroft, 2007).

Endocarditis

Endocarditis is common in adult pigs. In the majority of cases it is caused by *Erysipelothrix rhusiopathiae*, although on rare occasions other bacteria e.g. *Streptococcus* spp. are isolated. The clinical signs will vary depending on the valves involved. The severity will depend on the volume of the lesion. Initially there will be pyrexia. This may well subside with antibiotic treatment, e.g. injectable penicillin daily for 2 weeks. Normally the other clinical signs e.g. respiratory distress or peripheral oedema will persist, but in rare cases the condition will resolve. If this occurs it is advisable to give further antibiotics over the next parturition.

Eperythrozoon suis disease

This rickettsial parasite is seen in the UK and Europe but is much more common in the USA. It is spread by lice and by needles, but is also spread directly between pigs and spread from the sow to its piglets.

Often the condition is subclinical but it can cause weakness, anaemia and jaundice in piglets and growing pigs. It may cause acute pyrexia in fat pigs which may result in death. Anaemia and jaundice will be shown on post-mortem. The organism has been responsible for early embryonic loss in sows. The organism can be seen on Giemsa-stained blood smears. There is a PCR available.

Treatment is with oxytetracyclines. These can be injected as a long-acting preparation or given orally for 2 weeks. Some authorities recommend incorporation of chlorotetracycline into the food. This has not been helpful in the author's experience. When problems occur specifically in young piglets a single long-acting injection can be given 1 week before farrowing. Naturally, lice should be controlled.

Iron deficiency

This is a disease of piglets born to sows indoors, particularly in extremely clean units. The need for iron injections in newborn piglets is so well known that it is normally factored into the management system. However, mistakes can be made either with a whole litter being left out or individual piglets missing their iron injection.

The signs do not normally appear until 10 days of age. The piglets will be lethargic and visibly anaemic. They often have diarrhoea and show dyspnoea before dying. They will often die when stressed, so great care should be given when injecting them with iron. On post-mortem they will be very pale and even jaundiced. The heart will be enlarged and flabby. Often there is pericarditis. The diagnosis may be made on the post-mortem picture linked with the history. For confirmation, a blood haemoglobin level of <7 g/dl is diagnostic.

Lymphosarcoma

As this condition may be inherited it is reasonable to expect it to be sporadic, but in certain herds the incidence is too high. It is thought to be caused by an autosomal recessive gene. It can affect any age of growing pigs. It is not seen in adults.

The pigs will not thrive and there is lymph node enlargement which will cause differing signs depending on the lymph nodes involved. If the lymph nodes in the neck and mediastinum are involved there will be dyspnoea. Often the piglets appear to be 'poppy eyed'. Post-mortems will show generalized lymph node swellings. Histology will confirm the diagnosis. There is no treatment so euthanasia is advised. If a single boar can be implicated it should be culled.

Monensin poisoning

This drug can cause toxicity in pigs in three different scenarios.

1. The pigs are given monensin in their diet as a treatment for coccidiosis or some other pathogen.
2. The pigs are given access to cattle feed containing monensin in error.
3. The pigs are given access to medicated poultry feed in error.

Any oral level of 20 mg monensin/kg is liable to cause toxic signs. Death normally follows diarrhoea, dyspnoea and ataxia. There may be myoglobinuria and so the urine will be reddish brown. There is no treatment and euthanasia is indicated.

Mulberry heart disease

This disease is linked with hepatosis dietetica. Both are forms of vitamin E and selenium deficiency but the direct aetiology is not clear, nor is the link to muscular dystrophy. Mulberry heart disease can occur in all ages of pig but the most commonly affected age group is the fattening pig, particularly if it is growing really rapidly. The condition is extremely rarely seen in pigs fed a properly prepared ration. It is more commonly seen in farm-prepared rations or in backyard pigs fed straight cereals. Barley treated with proprionic acid is definitely a trigger factor for the disease which may reach epidemic proportions.

The best pigs in the group are affected and will often be found dead. Other pigs will be cyanotic, dyspnoeic with subnormal temperatures. The pulse is said to be rapidly raised with exercise and slow to return to normal. However the author has found this to be difficult to evaluate. Certainly stressful situations are liable to cause sudden death.

The post-mortem picture will be that of congestive heart failure. There will be an enlarged liver with a nutmeg appearance. There will be petichial haemorrhages under the epicardium and endocardium. There will be an excess of pericardial, pleural and peritoneal fluid. The definitive diagnosis will be reached by demonstrating low levels of vitamin E and selenium in the diet.

Some authorities suggest treatment should be given with vitamin E and selenium either orally or by injection to the whole group. This is a hazardous procedure as the stress will possibly cause more deaths. The author advises immediate supplementation of the diet with adequate levels of vitamin E and selenium, and treating only the anorexic pigs with injections of vitamin E and selenium. For further control there should be strict supplementation of the diet with vitamin E and selenium.

Hepatosis dietetica is normally seen in young growing pigs, i.e. a younger age group from animals showing mulberry heart disease. Animals may be found dead or *in extremis* with vomiting ataxia and jaundice. On post-mortem the liver may be pale or haemorrhagic but histologically the findings are pathognomonic.

Treatment is vitamin E and selenium. It is safe to give these by injection as stress does not normally lead to death, unlike the case in mulberry heart disease.

Muscular dystrophy can occur in mulberry heart disease or in hepatosis dietetica. Muscular dystrophy can occur in all ages of growing and fattening pigs. Affected animals will be lame and if examined carefully may show swelling of the large muscles of the limbs. These swollen muscles will be painful. Serum samples will show raised creatinine kinase (CK) levels. Treatment is injections of vitamin E and selenium together with NSAIDs.

Navel bleeding

At birth the umbilicus appears fatter than normal and tends to bleed. It may be a physical deformity which may be inherited. Various other causes have been suggested:

- Vitamin K deficiency.
- Vitamin C deficiency.
- Prostaglandin injection to bring on parturition.
- Sawdust or wood shavings used as bedding.

There is no evidence that any of these causes are connected, and in the author's experience vitamin C or K supplementation of the diet does not lessen the incidence of the condition. Equally, avoidance of prostaglandin injections or sawdust/wood shavings as bedding does not seem to improve the situation. The individual navels should be clamped using small plastic clamps marketed for the condition. 'Outbreaks' seem to stop. However it is prudent to check to see if one boar is involved.

Nitrite/nitrate poisoning

Nitrate is converted by the intestine into nitrite, which actually causes the toxicity. The likely source is slurry or when whey is fed. Nitrite causes haemoglobin to be converted into methaemoglobin. If the level of the latter exceeds the former by more than 75% death will occur from anoxia. Before these levels are reached the pigs will be lethargic, cyanotic and dyspnoeic. On post-mortem the blood appears chocolate in colour. A definitive diagnosis can be made by assaying the blood for methaemoglobin.

The recognized treatment is methylene blue given iv at a dose of 2 mg/kg. This is extremely difficult to accomplish in small pigs. The author has succeeded in affected sows by injecting into large superficial veins running above the mammary gland.

Pericarditis

This condition as a single entity is almost never seen in pigs. However, it is often seen linked with inflammation of other serous surfaces, e.g. pleurisy, peritonitis and arthritis in Glasser's disease.

Streptococcal lymphadenitis

Streptococcus porcinus has been isolated from the abscesses associated with the cervical lymph nodes in Eastern Europe and historically in the USA. The disease is seen in growing and fattening pigs and may not be apparent until the pigs are examined after slaughter. Infection occurs by contact. There is a vaccine available in some countries. Antibiotic medication can be used in the water or food after weaning.

Thiamin deficiency

This condition is rare in pigs. The author has seen it in pigs in a rescue sanctuary fed solely on waste bread from a supermarket. It is also said to occur in outdoor pigs kept on heath land and eating large quantities of bracken. Pigs are normally found dead. Post-mortem will reveal myocardial degeneration. There will be excess pericardial and pleural fluid. Thiamin can be injected im daily for 3 days. There is normally a good response to treatment.

Von Willebrand's disease

This is a haemophilia type of disease but is not sex linked. Clotting times are seriously prolonged. Often the condition is seen after iron injections. It is caused by an autosomal recessive gene.

Warfarin poisoning

Warfarin when used as a rat poison can cause poisoning in pigs. It is attractive to pigs and will be readily consumed. Normally the amount ingested will not be sufficient to poison a pig. However large quantities will cause pallor and haemorrhages. There will be vomiting and coughing blood. The treatment is large doses of vitamin K (20 mg vitamin K_1 per piglet im).

10 Diseases of the Urino-genital System

Urinary Problems

Nephritis/cystitis complex

The predominant sign will be either blood or pus in the urine. Urine can be collected in a clean sterile container for examination for blood, crystals and bacteria. Owners should be told not to use jam jars as there is likely to be sugar found erroneously in the sample. There is likely to be bacterial contamination even with a sterile container, so the results of culture should be judged with caution. The most likely modes of infection are parturition and service. Haematogenous infection of the kidneys is possible but is likely to be rare. The condition may be a low-grade local infection or a systemic infection with the pig showing a raised rectal temperature, lethargy and inappetence. If the infection is in the bladder, i.e. cystitis, the animal will be constantly passing small quantities of urine. Cystitis is much more common in sows than in boars. Pyelonephritis, an infection of the kidneys, is also more common in sows when caused by an ascending infection (Fig. 10.1). If pyelonephritis is caused by a haematogenous spread it is equally common in boars and sows.

Urinary infections are normally caused by *Actinobaculum suis*, *Escherichia coli* or *Klebsiella* spp. These organisms are commonly found in the prepuce of boars and in sows' vaginas, not causing clinical disease. As stated earlier their appearance in urine must be judged with caution. If found, particularly in pure culture, together with clinical disease they are likely to be significant. In these instances antibiotic sensitivity testing is well worthwhile. It is not known why in certain cases the infection is not killed by the sow's immune mechanisms. The rectal temperature is rarely raised initially when there is only cystitis, but it will become raised when the organism ascends the ureter and infects the kidney.

With appropriate prolonged antibiotic treatment the condition may be cured, or if only one kidney is infected the sow can appear to respond only to suffer relapses of the infection. She is obviously infectious to the boar. As the infection is in the urinary system she may come regularly into oestrus and may even get pregnant. In these cases it is prudent to inject a suitable antibiotic at farrowing to try to avoid a flare-up of the condition.

If several cases occur in a herd then routine treatment with antibiotics of both boars and sows before service may be justified. The author's preference is long-acting oxytetracycline given by injection at the appropriate time before service in the boar and after service in the sow. If antibiotics are given in the feed or water to all animals in the service area, the danger of antibiotic resistance is high.

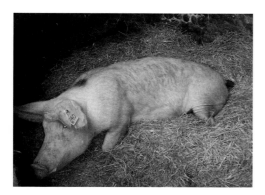

Fig. 10.1. A sow with pyelonephritis.

Porcine dermatitis and nephropathy syndrome

Porcine dermatitis and nephropathy syndrome (PDNS) is a serious condition which is mainly restricted to fattening pigs. It may even be seen at the abattoir with the stress of the journey bringing on the condition. Pigs may die rapidly and the condition may resemble CSF. Clinicians should consult more experienced colleagues if there is any doubt as to the diagnosis. There is a syndrome called 'rotting prepuce syndrome' which may be part of the PDNS condition. It occurs in entire boars. The ventral surface of the prepuce appears to be abraded. Some authorities have linked the condition to bedding on wheat straw. There may be actual necrosis not only to the prepuce but also to the abdominal wall. If it reaches an advanced state euthanasia is indicated, but in less severe cases antibiotics and NSAIDs by injection and oily creams topically may be beneficial. PDNS is also covered in the skin disease section (see Chapter 12).

Stephanurus dentatus

This is called the kidney worm. It does not occur in the UK but it is seen in tropical areas of North and South America. The worm uses earthworms as a secondary host. The adult worm, which is 2 mm in length, lives in the ureters and often causes nephritis. The eggs are shed in the urine and eaten by earthworms. When the earthworms are eaten by the pig the eggs turn into larvae and migrate through the liver, causing damage often seen at slaughter very similar to 'milk spot' caused by ascarid migration. They may also cause liver abscesses. The larvae find their way in the bloodstream to the ureters. The prepatent period is approximately 9 months. Ivermectin by injection is effective in eliminating larvae and adults.

Urolithiasis

This is caused by deposits of calcium carbonate. The reason for the deposits is unclear. It may be related to the diet. It is not related to a shortage of drinking water as this will cause salt poisoning as explained in the section covering neurological diseases (see Chapter 11). Urolithiasis is seen in sows and neonatal pigs. It is extremely rare in store pigs and is rare in finishing pigs. It can be prevented by providing a good diet. Treatment is difficult if there is a blockage of the urethra. In the author's experience this never occurs in sows as the urethra is large and is very easily catheterized, using a mare's urinary catheter. A blockage of the urethra is a disaster in a boar or a castrated boar as in the author's experience it is impossible to catheterize a male pig of any age even under a GA. In theory a urethrostomy could be performed below the anus provided the blockage is distal to this site. In reality euthanasia should be performed on welfare grounds.

Breeding and Reproductive Medicine for Commercial and Smallholder Pigs

Introduction

Reproductive management is not easy for smallholder pig owners. However, with normal vigilance they should be able to recognize oestrus and, by applying pressure to the back of the sow, should be able to detect standing oestrus. AI is not a difficult procedure in pigs. It has many advantages for the smaller breeder:

- There is no need to keep a boar, thus saving the capital outlay not only of the boar but also of the extra building and pens required. There are reduced feed costs, if a boar is not kept.

- Disease control is much easier if boars are not borrowed.
- New blood is easily introduced rather than keep changing boars.
- Safety is also important as often children are given access to smallholder pigs.

Reproductive biology

Pigs normally reach puberty at 6 months. However it should be noted that in pet pigs in a domestic environment and with the absence of other pigs, this may well be delayed. If after several months in a breeding situation, a sow or gilt does not show any evidence of oestrus, then hormonal means should be tried (see below). In a commercial situation, of course no special methods should be used before a sow or gilt has been allowed close contact with an active fertile boar.

The length of gestation is 114 days, with a normal variation of 2 days. The breeding cycles occur all year round, with oestrus occurring every 21 days with a variation of 1 day. The number of piglets per litter is very variable. It is affected not only by the genetics of the female but also the age of the female. After six litters the litter size tends to diminish.

Artificial insemination

To carry out AI commercial staff and smallholders require training. This can be obtained at agricultural colleges and from AI centres. Equipment is required which also can be obtained from AI centres. Naturally AI centres will have semen available from top sires and from most common breeds. If semen is required from a rare breed or an exotic breed then this should be ordered in advance.

Semen can be obtained from the Irelands AI centre:

Deerpark Pedigree Pigs
2 Drumanee Road
Bellaghy
Magherafelt

BT45 8LE
Tel: +44 (0)28 7938 6558

If orders are placed before 1 pm semen will arrive the next day.

Measures to aid reproduction

Oestrus can be synchronized by the use of oral altrenogest (see Appendix under Altresyn and Regumate porcine) in both gilts and sows. Gilts and sows will be expected to come into oestrus 5–7 days after the final day of administration of the drug. This same drug can be used to improve litter size in both gilts and sows. It can also be used to increase the farrowing rate in sows.

Parturition can be induced by 10 mg dinoprost given im within 3 days of expected parturition. Parturition can also be induced by 0.175 mg cloprostenol sodium given within 2 days of expected parturition. The use of either of these luteolytic agents to induce farrowing in sows and gilts will provide an opportunity for more efficient and convenient management under a variety of management systems. The advertised advantages are:

- Allows batch management of sows and gilts to be efficiently achieved.
- Minimizes farrowings at weekends, public holidays and during the night.
- Facilitates supervision of farrowing.
- Facilitates interfostering.
- Enables farrowing and labour schedules to be planned for convenience.
- Prevents sows and gilts going beyond term.
- Allows optimal use of farrowing quarters, equipment, etc.

To reduce the weaning to oestrus interval (WOI) and weaning to fertile service interval (WFSI) in sows in herds with reproductive problems, prostaglandin $F_{2\alpha}$ ($PGF_{2\alpha}$) has a stimulating effect on uterine contractions, leading to better postpartum evacuation of the uterus. Field clinical trials in herds with reproductive problems confirmed that treatment with 10 mg dinoprost at weaning resulted in a more rapid return to oestrus and fertile service after farrowing.

If gilts do not show signs of oestrus they may be induced to cycle by injections of hormones. Gilts over the age of 5 months will normally have a fertile oestrus within 5 days of an injection of 400 IU serum gonadotrophin and 200 IU chorionic gonadotrophin.

Sows post-weaning, particularly where early weaning is practised, if given an injection of 400 IU serum gonadotrophin and 200 IU chorionic gonadotrophin within 48 h of weaning, will result in an early postpartum oestrus.

Sows 40 days postpartum suffering from anoestrus post-weaning can be given 1000 IU serum gonadotrophin (pregnant mare serum gonadotrophin (PMSG)). This normally results in a fertile oestrus in 3–7 days.

Factors which affect reproductive performance

Haemoglobin (Hb) concentration decreases over time during the sow's productive life (Normand *et al.*, 2012). Gilts begin their reproductive life with a concentration of nearly 120 g/l; subsequent gestations appear to contribute to a decrease in Hb concentration, which falls below 110 g/l for sows of parity rank six or higher. Hb concentrations at farrowing and at weaning are lower than those measured 7 weeks before term. The thinner the sow, the lower is its Hb concentration, regardless of parity rank.

Pregnancy diagnosis

With commercial pigs the easiest method of pregnancy diagnosis is by noting whether the sow or gilt returns to oestrus at the next cycle (18–25 days); this is 85% accurate. However, in a smallholder situation or when there is a single pet sow the accuracy of this method falls to less than 50%. The external physical signs of pregnancy are fairly obvious in gilts after 60 days. The signs include: mammary development, enlargement of the abdomen and swelling of the vulva. The signs in sows are not reliable until about 3 weeks before term. Rectal palpation is not practical for

most veterinarians unless they have exceptionally small hands and the sow is large. After 60 days, pregnancy will be fairly obvious on rectal examination.

Historically, pulse echo and Doppler ultrasonography were used for pregnancy diagnosis. However, these have been superseded by real-time transabdominal ultrasonography, which can be accurate after 22 days using a sector head, although it is best carried out after 45 days using a linear bovine transrectal probe. Either way the probe is held low down on the flank just above the mammary line, just cranial to the hind leg.

Vaginal biopsy can be accurate after 36 days and is easy to perform if the sow is adequately restrained in a crate and if the correct biopsy tool, a 20 cm side-cutting vaginal probe, is used. The vulva is cleaned with chlorohexidine before the instrument is inserted along the dorsal wall of the vagina. A 12 mm segment of vaginal mucosa is removed and placed in formal saline. This is then sent to a suitable commercial laboratory.

In theory, blood oestrone sulfate levels after 35 days should be high enough to give a positive result of pregnancy. There is no laboratory doing these tests routinely in the UK at the time of writing, which makes the test very expensive.

Problems at Parturition

Abnormalities of parturition

There are more problems with parturition in pet pigs than in commercial pigs. This is not because there is anything intrinsically wrong with the breeds kept by smallholders, but because the owners fuss over them too much at term so that they forget the animal is a pig and fail to go through the normal hormonal pathways to initiate a correct farrowing sequence. If a clinician is called to an abnormal farrowing whether in a commercial or a pet sow, a vaginal examination should be performed if possible, with a well-lubricated gloved hand. Restraint may well be a problem. The provision of a farrowing crate to restrain the sow for examination is highly recommended.

The scenarios likely to be encountered are:

- The first stage of labour has not been accomplished. The sow or gilt should be left alone and then revisited in approximately 4 h. At that stage, if there have been no further developments the sow should be given an injection of prostaglandin.
- The second stage of labour has been reached but the cervix is not fully dilated. The rectal temperature should be checked for pyrexia and the mammary glands should be checked for any abnormalities. If any are found or there is pyrexia, then the animal should be given antibiotics and NSAIDs. If all appears normal the animal should be given an injection of prostaglandin and revisited in 4 h. If at that time there has been no further action, then a very small dose of oxytocin (2 IU) should be given im.
- If a piglet can be felt through the cervix, this should be drawn with gentle traction. There are polythene gloves available with small cord loops attached to the fingers, which can be useful if just the head of the piglet can be felt. Another small dose of oxytocin and antibiotics should be given.

Relative piglet oversize is extremely rare. The other problems likely to be encountered on rare occasions are a piglet stuck with its head in one horn and its hindquarters in the other horn and uterine torsion (see below). Hydrops allantois is an extremely rare condition in sows. The author has never seen the condition in the UK, only in Vietnam (Fig. 10.2).

Vaginal prolapse

This will occur before parturition, normally in the last few days of gestation which is likely to be 114 days. Sows should be given antibiotics and NSAIDs. With the sow in a crate, local anaesthetic should be injected around the vulva. A 'Buhner suture' should be placed in the vulva. This is best placed before replacing the vulva, so that as soon as the vulva is replaced the suture can be tightened. It is difficult to place the suture while retaining the vagina or worse, the cervix inside the sow.

To place a 'Buhner suture' the practitioner requires a long seaton needle, ideally 20–25 cm in length, and a 40 cm length of uterine tape. The point of the sharp needle is inserted ventrally directly below the vulva and then carefully directed dorsally between the skin and the left lip of the vulva to emerge

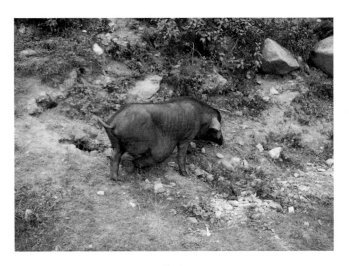

Fig. 10.2. Hydrops allantois in a Vietnamese Pot Bellied sow.

directly ventral to the anus. The uterine tape is threaded into the needle and it is withdrawn, leaving a single length of tape running from the anus subcutaneously to the ventral end of the vulva. The needle is re-inserted 0.5 cm to the right of the tape on the ventral end of the vulva and the process is repeated on the right side. The two ends of the tape will then be hanging down from the ventral end of the vulva. The vagina or the cervix and the vagina are replaced. The suture is then tightened so that only three fingers can be placed in the vulva. The suture is then tied with a bow, so that if the pig keeper thinks the sow is farrowing he or she can undo the suture without cutting it. If the sow is actually farrowing he/she can let her farrow and then retie the suture when the sow is finished; but if the sow is not farrowing the suture can be retied immediately before the vagina prolapses again.

When farrowing is complete the suture should be left in place for 48 h and then removed. The sow should receive antibiotics and NSAIDs daily until the suture is removed. This condition is almost certain to recur at subsequent farrowings and so the sow should not be served again.

Uterine torsion

This condition is seen in parturient pigs but it is extremely rare. The only reported instance was by the author. A total torsion of the uterus will be seen. Diagnosis is simple as the rifling of the vagina will be felt on vaginal examination. The sow should be given a GA as described in Chapter 6 and placed in lateral recumbency with her right side on the ground if the rifling is in a clockwise direction or on her left side if the rifling is in an anticlockwise direction. The sow should then be rolled over on to her back quickly in the direction of the rifling. On re-examination per vagina the twist should have gone and any piglets within reach can be removed. Until parturition is complete 10 IU of oxytocin can be injected im at 30 min intervals so that the piglets can be removed. Antibiotics and NSAIDs should be given. If the twist has not gone the procedure can be repeated once.

If it is still not successful a Caesarean section should be carried out.

Torsion of one horn of the uterus is more common. The author recorded 34 cases in a period of 15 years' full-time mixed practice with a 25% pig practice workload. The presenting history is a sow passing several pigs and some afterbirth and then parturition will cease. This is likely to be the total number of pigs in the single normally positioned horn. The torsion of the abnormal horn is felt on a full vaginal and cervical examination. Rolling should not be attempted. Humane destruction was requested in 32 cases. A Caesarean section was carried out in two cases.

Farrowing fever complex

This is the most common problem found in parturient pigs. There are multiple presenting signs. These are: a slow parturition, inappetence, constipation, a hard painful udder, a failure to pass all the afterbirths and pyrexia. The latter is common but is not an invariable finding.

A full clinical examination should be performed. The rectal temperature will normally be raised initially but this will often drop to a subnormal temperature as the disease progresses. Palpation of the udder will often reveal a hot, swollen, hard mammary gland. This indication of an acute mastitis will be shown in the majority of cases but is not an invariable sign. A vaginal examination may reveal piglets which will normally be dead and/or afterbirth. Any dead piglets and afterbirth should be removed. The most likely pathogen is *E. coli*. If there is a slow parturition, there is an injectable solution of vetrabutine hydrochloride which is licensed for use in sows as a specific uterine relaxant and musculotropic stimulator. This drug dilates the soft birth canal and coordinates uterine contractions to ease and shorten parturition. Vetrabutine may also be useful in cases of dystocia where there is insufficient relaxation of the birth canal.

Farrowing fever complex is a syndrome which has been called mastitis, metritis, agalactia syndrome (MMA). This description can be misleading because it assumes that all three clinical signs are always present. In the author's experience this is rarely the case. If parturition is slow or if there has been considerable human intervention the main sign will be metritis. This will require specific treatment for metritis which may be different from the treatment for mastitis and even for less specific agalactia.

MMA has received a large amount of coverage in both the veterinary literature and the lay pig press. It is sometimes termed 'milk fever'. This is unwise as it is totally different from 'milk fever' which is so common in dairy cattle. It is NOT hypocalcaemia which is not a feature in parturient pigs. Calcium borogluconate should never be administered to pigs as it causes a severe reaction if administered sc.

MMA is normally the result of an *E. coli* infection that affects the mammary gland and the uterus soon after parturition. It is normally associated with a slow farrowing. A streptococcal or staphylococcal metritis may also be involved, particularly after human intervention. In many cases the condition can be prevented by prompt treatment with a penicillin/streptomycin mixture being given im for 3 days following any human intervention.

Agalactica may be part of the complex as the name suggests. However it may also be caused by a lack of exercise and the resulting constipation. A laxative diet prior to farrowing is obviously beneficial.

For treatment of MMA a suitable antibiotic together with an NSAID should be injected. The choice of antibiotic has been given considerable debate: if the main organism is a *Streptococcus* sp., penicillin is the drug of choice, particularly as it gives high levels in the uterus. If a *Staphylococcus* sp. (and particularly a penicillin-resistant *Staphylococcus* sp.) is involved, synthetic penicillins with or without clavulanic acid will be worthwhile. These will also be effective if the main problem is *E. coli* in the udder. Some authorities recommend oral tetracyclines; they are particularly useful in smallholder and pet pigs where repeated daily injections should be avoided. Tetracyclines are very well absorbed by pigs in a water-soluble solution as a follow-up to the injection. Historically,

practitioners used to give dexamethazone to reduce the inflammation in the mammary gland. With the advent of NSAIDs the author would recommend them rather than dexamethazone. NSAIDs and dexamethazone certainly should not be given at the same time. Oxytocin is a useful drug either if parturition is complete or if there is a likelihood of further pigs being born. In this latter case it should be given as small intramuscular doses of 5 IU, with vaginal examinations being repeated at 6 h intervals. If parturition is complete 30 IU can be given as a single intramuscular dose.

Liquid paraffin at the rate of 500 ml/day per sow on the surface of the water will help with any constipation. Trying to administer liquids to adult pigs by mouth by any other means is not easy.

Caesarean section

Rarely in a commercial situation is a Caesarean section justifiable economically. However, in pet pig practice it may be requested when there is an uncorrectable uterine torsion. Welfare must always be considered. If the piglets are still alive and the handling facilities are adequate then a Caesarean section may be appropriate. The sow should be given a GA (see Chapter 6). When the sow is in lateral recumbency the upper hind leg should be drawn back with a rope, so that the incision can be made as caudal as possible. The area from the hind leg forward including the mammary glands and half the flank should be cleaned. As the GA is unlikely to last long enough to totally complete the Caesarean section, local infiltration should be carried out for a 25 cm incision in a para-medium position just above the mammary gland. It is hoped that even if the sow is recovering from the GA, with this local anaesthesia she will remain in lateral recumbency. The area should be prepared for surgery. Antibiotics and NSAIDs should be given. A 20 cm incision should be made through the skin, muscle layers and peritoneum, 1 cm above the mammary gland as far caudal as possible. The body of the uterus should be brought up to the incision. A 12 cm incision should be made into the body of the uterus, or if there is a torsion of one horn then the incision should be made in this horn. An assistant should hold up either side of the uterus up to the abdominal incision with two pairs of uterine forceps. All piglets and their afterbirths should be removed from the uterus and the piglets should be placed in a warm box. A very careful examination should be made to make sure ALL of the piglets are removed. The uterus should then be closed with a single continuous row of Lembert sutures with absorbable suture material. Some antibiotics should be applied along the suture line and into the abdomen. In the case of a torsion, the uterus should be returned to the correct orientation and position. 30 IU oxytocin should be given im. The abdominal musculature including the peritoneum should be sutured with two rows of continuous mattress sutures using absorbable suture material.

The skin should then be sutured with single horizontal mattress sutures. Number 1 polypropylene material on a swaged 48 mm, 12.5 mm reverse cutting needle is very suitable for this task. These skin sutures need to be very close together as the piglets may try to interfere with them when suckling. The piglets should be encouraged to suckle. Antibiotics and NSAIDs should be given for a minimum of 5 days.

Problems after Parturition

Vaginal discharge and/or metritis

This is a common sequel to parturition and will lead to the farrowing fever syndrome described above. It may also occur after mating. The old-fashioned approach of inserting pessaries is now thought not to be appropriate. Treatment should be antibiotics and oxytocin by injection. If metritis has occurred after mating then sexual rest should be maintained until 2 weeks after all vulval discharge has ceased. Boars may transmit infection. Although penile infection is rarely seen, preventive treatment of the boar with parenteral antibiotics is of value. Local treatment with antibiotics into the sheath has been

suggested; this is difficult to do, however, and probably best avoided.

Uterine prolapse

This is a very serious problem (Fig. 10.3). Practitioners must consider the welfare issues as recovery rates are not good, particularly if the prolapse is older than 3 h or if handling facilities are not good. Euthanasia should be carried out if practitioners are in any doubt of reasonable chances of recovery. In commercial pigs euthanasia is the best economic option. In the case of pet pigs, if there is a live litter then treatment should be attempted.

The sow should be given a GA (see Chapter 6) and also given antibiotics and NSAIDs by injection. The sow should be hoisted in a farrowing crate and have her hocks tied to either side of the top of the crate. A conventional straw bale should be placed under her hindquarters so that her head and forequarters are low down at the front of the crate. The prolapsed uterus should be placed on a clean polythene sack on the straw bale. The uterus should be checked for any damage. If there is damage to the uterine wall, it should be sutured with horizontal mattress sutures of absorbable material making sure the peritoneal surfaces are opposed. The vulva should be lubricated before pushing one hand gently into the tip of one uterine horn and slowly replace it into the sow. When the tip is well over the pelvic brim a flicking motion together with gravity will make the

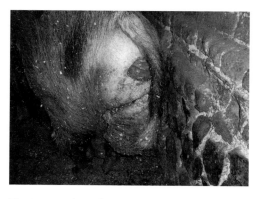

Fig. 10.3. Prolapsed uterus.

uterine horn descend into the correct position. The process should be repeated with the second horn and the body of the uterus. After the practitioner is satisfied that the uterus has been returned to its correct position, the vulva should be closed with a 'Buhner suture'. 30 IU of oxytocin should be injected im. Antibiotics and NSAIDs should be continued for two further days, when the 'Buhner suture' can be removed.

Chronic mastitis

One or more mammary glands will be large, swollen and non-productive. They are rarely painful and the sow does not appear to be ill or have pyrexia. The condition may be caused by a variety of organisms, usually *Arcanobacterium pyogenes*. Antibiotic treatment, even if prolonged, will not be effective. The gland should not be lanced. If the gland ulcerates humane destruction should be carried out. If the gland does not burst and the sow is kept for subsequent breeding, it is prudent to give antibiotics in a preventive manner at subsequent farrowings in the hope of preventing further glands becoming infected.

Abortions, Stillbirths, Weak and Mummified Piglets

Introduction

There are very many causes of abortions, stillbirths, weak and mummified piglets. Nearly all infectious or toxic causes will cause all of these manifestations. It is the time in the pregnancy when the agent or toxin affects the sow that will determine which of these problems will occur. Thus, if the agent affects the sow in the first five weeks of pregnancy, there is likely to be a vulval discharge with a subsequent return to service. If the agent affects the sow between the sixth and eighth week of pregnancy some or all of the piglets are likely to be mummified at term. If the agent affects the sow after the eighth week of pregnancy there is likely to be abortion, stillbirths or weak piglets at term. It should be remembered that

any disease causing a fever might cause an abortion. So-called 'barker' piglets are thought to be just a manifestation of prematurity.

The cause of a single abortion is rarely found. Less than 10% of abortions where both the fetus and the afterbirth are submitted to the laboratory have the causal organism isolated. With multiple abortions the diagnostic rate from retrospective serum samples is rarely as high as 20%.

Common causes of abortion, stillbirths, weak and mummified piglets

African swine fever

The ASF virus, which causes high temperatures, will cause abortions not only because the virus may target the uterus but also because the high temperatures experienced by the sow will cause abortion. It should be remembered that this is a notifiable disease.

Aujeszky's disease

This viral disease used to be called pseudorabies. It should be remembered that this is a notifiable disease in the UK. It is likely to cause 100% mortality in newly born piglets and 60% in older piglets. These piglets are likely to show neurological signs before death. There may be few signs in adult sows except abortion and small herpes cold sore-type lesions on the snout. The aborted piglets will have necrotic foci in their livers and in their spleens. Necrotic lesions will be seen in the placentae. Histological sections of liver, spleen and placentae will show pathognomic inclusion bodies.

Blue eye paramyxovirus

This virus causes abortions in parts of Mexico. It is possible that the virus occurs in mainland Europe and in Northern Ireland (Stephano *et al.*, 1988). It has not been isolated in the last 20 years. The virus is similar to human 'mumps'.

Brucellosis

Brucella suis has not been recorded in the UK or Eire and is not notifiable, but is reportable under the Zoonosis Order 1989. It is found on mainland Europe with hares and wild boars as potential reservoirs. It is also recorded in the USA. In areas where the organism is found surveillance is carried out by sampling submissions of abortion material and pigs with a history of lameness and/or paralysis are cultured. Although serological tests are used, they are not considered specific enough for individual screening of pigs. Pigs imported into AI centres from Officially Brucellosis Free (OBF) countries are tested for brucellosis, as are boars producing semen in these centres on an annual basis.

Brucellosis in pigs can occasionally be associated with synovitis and hygromas leading to lameness, inco-ordination and posterior paralysis, as well as reproductive signs. Abortions may not be widespread but there will be signs of orchitis in boars and a severe endometritis in sows.

There are numerous validated assays used for the detection of antibodies produced in response to the classical *Brucella*, yet no single test can be expected to identify every infected animal (Millar and Stack, 2012). The Rose Bengal plate test (RBPT) is a cheap, simple agglutination test commonly used for surveillance purposes in the UK and worldwide. Positive results are further checked with other serological tests, including ELISA and the complement fixation test (CFT).

False positive serological reactions are common in brucellosis serological tests and are caused by antibodies produced in response to infections with bacteria such as *Yersinia enterocolitica* 0:9, which is particularly common in pigs.

Carbon monoxide

This poisonous gas can cause abortion. Fetal tissue will be cherry red. Pigs should not be kept in garages nor should tractors be run for any length of time in pig accommodation which is poorly ventilated.

Classical swine fever

CSF is a notifiable disease in the UK. There are highly virulent strains which will kill sows. There are less virulent strains which will cause abortion. There are good vaccines available but they are not permitted in the UK or in the USA.

Erysipelas

This condition may cause abortions on account of the high fever shown by some animals. It also may cause abortion as a pathogen. It is regularly found in aborted fetuses. It is the most common recorded cause of abortion in the UK. There is a good vaccine available. If aborted animals show high levels of antibodies and have not been vaccinated, that would give an indication that *Erysipelothrix rhusiopathiae* has caused the abortion.

Foot and mouth disease

This highly contagious viral disease, which is notifiable in the UK, will cause abortions in pigs. It should be considered as a cause of abortion in other parts of the world where it is endemic.

Japanese B encephalitis virus infection

Pigs amplify this zoonotic virus which is not found in the UK. It is found in India, the Far East and in Queensland, Australia. It is spread by mosquitoes. Diagnosis is by ELISA or RT-PCR. It will also affect boars. They will have low or zero sperm counts and will lack libido. Obviously infected boars should not be used for semen collection for AI. There is a live attenuated vaccine available, which should be given twice with an interval of 2 weeks to all breeding stock before the start of the mosquito season. There are also killed, oil adjuvanted vaccines available which can be used for continuous year-round cover.

Leptospirosis

There are eight *Leptospira* spp. which are relevant in pigs. They may cause inapparent infection but all of them have been implicated in causing abortions and stillbirths in pigs. They may also cause the sow to be ill but this is rare. They definitely will cause pyrexia, icterus and death in piglets. The incidence of the various species varies in different countries.

They also vary in incidence depending on whether the sows are housed or outdoors.

Leptospires are bacteria classified as spirochaetes. They are very sensitive to desiccation and most disinfectants but they will survive in water for long periods. Infection is normally by ingestion but can be venereally and even through cuts. They migrate to the kidney and are shed in the urine. They tend to cause abortion a month after infection. The organisms may remain in the reproductive tract of both sows and boars. Rats may spread the disease. Rats may infect pigs, dogs and man. Pigs may also infect man. The disease in man is normally restricted to farm workers, slaughtermen, veterinary surgeons and butchers.

Treatment of ill piglets should be injections of combinations of penicillin/streptomycin. Tiamulin can be used in the water. Abortions may be prevented by a single dose of streptomycin at 25 mg/kg. This can be used as a long-term preventative. Sows should be injected 1 week before service and again 2 weeks before farrowing. If animals are not infected they should be vaccinated with a killed vaccine containing the correct serotype before service. Piglets should be vaccinated at weaning. Feedback of fetal material advocated by some authors to control stillbirths, mummification, embryonic deaths and infertility (SMEDI) should be avoided as such practices will spread leptospirosis.

Mycotoxins

There is a variety of mycotoxins which will cause reproductive problems in pigs. Infection will mainly come from dirty food bins or food bags stored in damp conditions. The aborted or stillborn piglets will be seen to have enlarged teats. However, early embryonic death is a more common manifestation (see Chapter 15).

Porcine parvovirus

PPV really only causes reproductive disease, but has been implicated in poor growth rates of piglets and diarrhoea. It occurs worldwide. It is spread oro-nasally and venereally. It is found in semen. It may cause early fetal death

with resorption and return to service, but more commonly it causes mummification of piglets and abortion. The clinical history and findings will indicate a diagnosis. The diagnosis can be confirmed by PCR or ELISA. Serology is helpful only in unvaccinated animals. There is a very effective vaccine. It is important to vaccinate gilts and sows before service. Boars should also be vaccinated. Initially each animal requires two doses of killed vaccine. This will give an immunity of at least 2 years. After an abortion the sow will be immune.

Porcine circovirus infection

The type 2 virus which is ubiquitous will cause abortion. However it is not a primary cause of abortion in the UK. There is a vaccine available.

Porcine reproductive and respiratory syndrome

This disease is commonly called 'blue ear disease'. The acute respiratory disease is shown in growing pigs but it is very transitory in adults which will abort. It is a primary cause of abortion in the UK. There is a vaccine available.

Salmonella spp.

These bacteria cause pyrexia and abortions. Mainly the abortion is because of the pyrexia but sometimes the organism can be isolated from the placenta or the fetus.

Stillbirths, mummification, embryonic deaths and infertility

This syndrome (SMEDI) is caused by an enterovirus and is difficult to distinguish diagnostically from parvovirus. The virus can be isolated from frozen or chilled fetal lung. Paired serum samples are useful. Serology can be carried out on transudates from thoracic cavities of freshly dead piglets. There is no vaccine available, so isolation is really the only realistic measure for control. Some authorities advise the grinding up of faeces, fetal membranes and mummified fetuses and feeding this to the sows and gilts at least

3 weeks before service. This acts as a home-made vaccine. However this practice is contrary to the Waste Foods Order in the UK. It also is hazardous as it may spread many other diseases.

Swine influenza

This virus disease mainly causes respiratory signs but also causes pyrexia and abortions. It is not a primary cause of abortion in the UK. There is a vaccine available.

Toxoplasmosis

In theory this protozoal zoonosis, which is harboured by cats, might cause abortion in pigs. It has been confirmed only in isolated cases.

Vitamin A deficiency

This is an extremely rare condition and therefore it is an extremely rare cause of abortion in pigs. The author has only once seen the condition in backyard pigs receiving a very inappropriate, poorly balanced diet.

Seasonal Infertility

This is seen in temperate countries like the UK. It occurs in the summer particularly in those rare summers which have an extended period of warm weather. However, the cause may not be temperature but day length. Fertility in wild boars drops off as the day length becomes shorter. Certainly increasing artificial light, or rather, not allowing the day length to decrease in housed pigs helps fertility rates.

Hot weather in outdoor pigs seems to induce lethargy in both boars and sows. The provision of good shade and adequate wallows helps to prevent any drop in fertility in the summer months.

11 Diseases of the Neurological System

Neurological Conditions

Introduction

The importance of neurological conditions in pigs will relate to the purpose for which they are being kept. In commercial herds contagious and infectious neurological diseases are very important. In small pig herds management causes of neurological conditions, e.g. water deprivation leading to salt poisoning, will be important. Individual pet pigs kept until they are very old may suffer from brain tumours. Practitioners must have at the forefront of their minds that whatever type of pig is being examined may have neurological signs which are either primary or secondary to notifiable diseases.

The predominant signs

These are best observed before handling. They include: abnormalities of gait including high stepping, abnormal posture, aural discharge, circling, convulsions, facial paralysis, flaccid tail, head tilt, hyperaesthesia, lack of pedal withdrawal, loss of balance, mania, nystagmus, ocular discharge, opisthotonos, paddling, recumbency, stupor and tremor.

Diagnosis

This will rely on an accurate history and on accurate observation. Certain conditions will be age related. The condition of the skin and the rectal temperature will be useful.

Neurological Diseases Caused by Viruses

African swine fever

This is notifiable in the UK. The peracute nature of this disease may give rise to nervous signs but they are not a consistent feature. It is not normally classified as a neurological disease (see Chapters 13 and 14). It will also cause abortions.

Aujeszky's disease

This is notifiable in the UK (see Chapter 14). It is classified as a neurological disease. It was called pseudo-rabies in the past. The neurological signs are more prominent in baby pigs. It will also cause abortions. It used to occur worldwide but it has now been eradicated in the USA and most of Europe. It is still found in South-east Asia and South America.

It is caused by an alphaherpesvirus. There is only one major antigenic type recognized. The virus is sensitive to heat, lysol, formaldehyde, sodium hypochlorite and detergents.

The virus enters the pig via the upper respiratory tract and after multiplying travels up the olfactory nerves to the CNS. There is venereal spread. Some strains will cause respiratory disease. Animals will start shedding virus within 2 days of infection. This may continue for 3 weeks.

Morbidity and mortality may reach 100% in suckling piglets. Mortality in fattening pigs may be as high as 15%. Often adults show only mild pyrexia but 50% may abort. Normally mortality in adults is under 2%. The virus causes infertility in boars.

Often there are no gross pathological findings. In piglets there may be small petechiae in the lymph nodes and the kidney. There may be congestion in the meninges and an excess of CSF. There may be a few white necrotic foci in the tonsils. In the respiratory form there will be lung involvement. Boars may have one testicle enlarged. Aborted piglets will have yellow necrotic foci in the liver. The placentae may appear normal but histology will reveal necrotic lesions and inclusion bodies. The main histological findings are in the CNS.

The disease will spread with the introduction of carrier animals. It will also spread by aerosol for a mile or so. Greater distances have been recorded. It may be spread in semen, fomites and rodents. Wild boar may be a reservoir of infection. It may cause death in other species e.g. cats, dogs, sheep and cattle. Pruritis is marked in other species.

Diagnosis may be confirmed by FAT on frozen tonsil tissue. Serology will indicate past infection. Meat juice may be used as a screening test.

There are various live and dead vaccines available. They are not now used in the UK or in the rest of the EU or the USA.

Bovine spongiform encephalopathy

Bovine spongiform encephalopathy (BSE) has been experimentally induced in pigs but it cannot be transmitted by feeding either infected bovine brain or scrapie material obtained from sheep.

Classical swine fever

CSF is notifiable in the UK. As with ASF, the peracute nature of this virus disease may give rise to nervous signs particularly in baby piglets. It is not normally classified as a neurological disease (see Chapters 13 and 14). It will also cause abortions.

Eastern equine encephalitis

Outbreaks have been recorded of this neurological virus spread by mosquitoes in the south-eastern USA and Mexico. Mortality may be high in growing pigs. The main pathological signs are in the myocardium not in the CNS.

Japanese B encephalitis

This disease is caused by a flavivirus and is spread by mosquitoes. It is found in Asia and has spread to Queensland in Australia. It is a very sensitive virus and is rapidly inactivated by heat and disinfectants. The virus infects the pig from a mosquito bite. There is an immediate viraemia and the virus reaches the CNS. Piglets will die. Sows will abort and boars will lose libido and become infertile. Wild birds may be a reservoir and man may be infected (see Chapter 16). Diagnosis is with an ELISA or a RT-PCR. Infected boars should not be used. There is a live attenuated vaccine available. Adults should be vaccinated before the start of the mosquito season.

Rabies

This is a notifiable disease which is not likely to be seen in the UK. It is classified as a neurological disease. It is extremely rare in pigs even where rabies is endemic. Pigs do excrete the virus in their saliva, so practitioners should take care. The 'dumb' form of rabies with excessive salivation is the most common but the 'rage' form is also seen (see Chapter 14). It is caused by a ribonucleic acid (RNA) lyssavirus. It may have a long incubation period up to 4 months. Once clinical signs are apparent it is invariably fatal. Incubating animals have been saved by vaccination.

Swine vesicular disease

Encephalitis is seen in pigs with swine vesicular disease (SVD). It is not normally classified as a neurological disease. Young pigs will scream from pain when they move. The problem with the disease is that the lesions cannot be differentiated from FMD. Both diseases are notifiable in the UK (see Chapter 14).

Talfan disease

This is a notifiable disease which has been very rarely recorded in the UK. It is thought to be a mild form of Teschen disease. It is classified as a neurological disease. It is part of a group of diseases known as polioencephalomyelitis. It is mainly seen in piglets rather than older pigs. There is an ELISA test available.

Teschen disease

This is a notifiable disease which is classified as neurological disease but has never been recorded in the UK. It is seen in Central Europe. Marked pyrexia and severe neurological signs are seen. Pigs will be anorexic and show inco-ordination. This may be followed by tremors and convulsions. Pigs will become paralysed and die. There will be no gross pathological changes seen. However, neuronal degeneration will be seen in the grey matter on histological samples. There is an ELISA test available. Vaccination using a live attenuated vaccine is carried out in Central and Eastern Europe.

Neurological Diseases Caused by Bacteria and Their Treatment

Abscesses

If these occur in the spinal cord they are normally as a result of tail biting. The pig will be paraplegic. There is rarely pyrexia. They can occur in the brain as a result of haematological spread. The pig may then show a variety of neurological signs. They can show pyrexia. Large doses of antibiotics together with NSAIDs can be tried for treatment but it is rarely successful.

Actinobacillosis

This disease is caused by two organisms, *Actinobacillus suis* and *Actinobacillus equuili*. It is not classified as a neurological disease. There may be neurological signs in the peracute form in piglets up to 6 weeks of age. There is pyrexia, septicaemia, arthritis and endocarditis. In older pigs the disease is less acute with skin lesions and a necrotizing focal pneumonia. Adults may die with an endocarditis. Antibiotics given as a treatment are rarely successful but can be used to reduce the incidence of the disease (see Chapter 9).

Bowel oedema

This is really an enteric disease, not a neurological condition. The acute septicaemia can cause oedema of the CNS and so give neurological signs, but oedema of the eyelids will also be seen to aid diagnosis. Pigs should have their rations reduced and be given antibiotics in the water (see Chapter 8).

Haemophilus parasuis meningitis

This is part of the Glasser's disease syndrome. It is not a neurological disease per se. All the serous surfaces are affected including the meninges, so neurological signs can be a feature of this disease as well as respiratory signs. The disease is sporadic. Antibiotics are rarely useful for treatment (see Chapter 9).

Leptospirosis

Certain *Leptospira* spp. cause liver toxicity which results in jaundice. Affected animals may show neurological signs. Leptospirosis is not classified as a neurological disease. The antibiotic of choice for treatment is streptomycin. Practitioners should remember the zoonotic implications.

Listeriosis

This neurological disease is caused by *Listeria monocytogenes*. The organism has been found in normal pigs at slaughter. Deaths in neonatal pigs showing neurological signs have been recorded. It is an extremely rare disease in pigs. Diagnosis can be made on culture. Treatment and prevention can be attempted with oxytetracyclines.

Middle-ear infection

The main sign will be shaking of the head. This will result in the formation of aural haematomas in adult lop-eared breeds. The infection is likely to follow mange. Treatment must involve treating the sarcoptic mange as well as the secondary infection. Obvious aural haematomas may be treated as in dogs under a GA in a variety of surgical ways. In view of the dangers of anaesthetics in adult pigs, this procedure cannot be recommended. Equally practitioners should NOT be tempted to release the swelling by cutting the aural skin. The haemorrhage will be very significant and not appreciated by the pig owner. If the mites and the bacteria can be controlled, the head shaking will stop and the ear will heal as a 'cauliflower ear'.

Salmonellosis

This disease causes a high fever which may give neurological signs in young pigs. It is normally considered as an enteric disease not a neurological condition (see Chapter 8).

Streptococcal meningitis

This is one of the most common neurological diseases to affect pigs. It is caused by *Streptococcus suis* type 1. The most usual condition in the UK occurs in the 8–12 week age group. Pigs may be found dead, but the condition is more commonly seen as pigs which are unable to sit up and are paddling. They will have a raised rectal temperature. Antibiotics, normally penicillin, are very helpful. A small dose of dexamethasone will cut down the inflammation in the CNS. Survival will also be aided by supplying fluids by mouth. Care must be taken not to choke the pig. An old teapot is useful to pour a stream of water for the affected pig to lick. There is a much less common streptococcal condition in the UK shown in fat pigs which is called 'type 2 meningitis'. Pigs are normally found dead. 'Type 2' is more common in the rest of the world. If the pigs are not found dead they will have a very high rectal temperature. Joint ill may occur in 1- to 2-week-old pigs, which is caused by *S. suis*.

The disease, either the neurological form or the joint ill form, may become an epidemic. The disease is spread by contact or by aerosol. The diagnosis will be straightforward on clinical signs and PME. The organism can be seen on smears of heart blood or CSF and stained by Gram. There is a PCR available.

The first method of control should be to review the husbandry procedures. Overcrowding and poor ventilation should be avoided. Mixing of pigs from different litters should be reduced as much as possible. Ideally there should be an 'all-in all-out' policy. Animals should be reared in dry pens with as little slurry as possible and as low a humidity level as can be arranged.

There is no vaccine available at the time of writing. Eradication or slaughter and restocking are unlikely to be successful. There are various medication regimens recommended depending on when the pigs develop clinical signs. Injectable long-acting penicillin can be given strategically at birth, then 10 days after weaning; in fact at any stage if the disease is a problem. If water medication is required in pigs after weaning the author's preference is amoxicillin. Other authorities advise tilmicosin. This antibiotic can also be given in-feed. The author's preference for in-feed medication is procaine penicillin at 300 g/t.

Tetanus

This neurological disease is very rarely found in pigs as they are very resistant to the tetanus toxin. Routine antitoxin injections need not be given in this species. The pig will appear rigid with the tail sticking out. Penicillin maybe given but the clostridial bacteria are likely to be dead long before the symptoms appear. Recovery is normally complete over a 10-day period.

Neurological Diseases Caused by Protozoa

Coccidiosis

This is not a neurological disease. It may cause severe enteric signs in baby pigs. The dehydration may result in neurological signs.

Neurological Diseases of Newly Born Piglets

Barking piglets

These are piglets which are dysmature. They have domed heads and never breath properly. The resulting expiratory effort sounds like a bark. They die rapidly or they should be humanely destroyed.

Congenital meningoencephalocoele

This is an inherited condition and is recorded in Landrace and Large White pigs. It is an autosomal recessive condition. The meninges

can be seen through the top of the skull where the bones have not fused.

Congenital tremor AI

Piglets showing this tremor are born to sows which have suffered from CSF or have been vaccinated against CSF. Therefore the condition is not seen in the UK.

Congenital tremor AII

This is also called myoclonia congenita. It occurs worldwide. The adults are asymptomatic but an unknown infection or poison causes the piglets to be born with a tremor. If they do not shake too violently and can keep sucking on to a nipple they will survive. The condition does not occur to piglets in subsequent litters. Normally the outbreak will last about 4 months.

Congenital tremor AIII

This sex-linked recessive gene is seen only in male Landrace piglets.

Congenital tremor AIV

This is an inherited condition seen in Saddleback pigs. Boars should be changed as it will occur in subsequent litters. It also rarely occurs in Saddleback pigs crossed with Large White pigs.

Congenital tremor AV

If sows are exposed to trichlorfon or Neguvon® (mange treatments) during a period of their gestation from 6 to 11 weeks, trembling piglets will be born at term.

Congenital tremor type B

When there is no known cause for the birth of trembling piglets they are said to have type B congenital tremor.

Copper deficiency

Stillbirths and ataxic piglets have been recorded but this is an extremely rare condition.

Hypoglycaemia

This condition occurs when newborn piglets get hypothermic, i.e. in outdoor pigs. The first signs are ataxia followed by convulsions. It is vital that the piglets receive 15 ml of 5% w/w glucose ip BEFORE they are warmed up.

Splay leg

This condition of piglets is seen when sows have been fed mouldy rations containing the fungus *Fusarium*.

Vitamin A deficiency

This condition is extremely rare. Piglets born to deficient sows will be weak and show neurological signs. The condition is not reversible but can be prevented by feeding an adequate diet.

Neurological Disease Caused by Miscellaneous Causes

Heat stroke

This condition will certainly cause neurological signs. They are very similar to water deprivation (salt poisoning). Over-fat Vietnamese Pot Bellied Pigs are very susceptible. Sunburn may complicate the condition in white pigs. Pigs should be cooled rapidly with buckets of cold water or a hose. If they are *in extremis*, dexamethazone given iv will be helpful. If the pigs have sunburn they will require antibiotics, NSAIDs and topical oily creams.

12 Diseases of the Skin

Introduction

Lesions on the skin can be caused by systemic disease, e.g. FMD, PRRS, CSF, ASF, SVD and salmonellosis. Only actual skin disease will be covered in this chapter.

Skin Diseases Caused by Viruses

Swinepox

This is an extremely rare condition which can be congenital. The normal manifestation is multiple crusted pustules. The virus on its own is a mild condition unless it leads to a secondary condition, e.g. severe greasy pig disease. This more aggressive bacterial skin disease will need treatment. The virus condition is self-limiting and so there is no need for treatment. Swinepox is thought to be spread by lice and biting flies. Diagnosis is by virus isolation and retrospective serology. Herds rapidly gain immunity and so the condition will disappear unless naive pigs are brought on to the farm.

Skin Diseases Caused by Bacteria

Abscesses

These are common and normally follow wounds from fighting. They may also lead on from an initial haematoma which then becomes infected by haematogenous spread. A wide variety of bacteria may be isolated. These would include: *Streptococcus* spp., *Staphylococcus* spp., *Bacteriodes* spp. and *Arocanobacterium pyogenes*. Equally, they are often sterile. They may be seen as swellings anywhere on the body irrespective of age or gender (Fig. 12.1).

Differentiation from haematomata is not straightforward. In theory abscesses should be hard, hot and painful and haematomata should be soft, fluctuating and not really painful. Ultrasonography may be helpful but paracentesis is the ultimate diagnostic tool. It is very important that this is carried out in a sterile manner as haematomata are easily infected to become abscesses. The skin should be carefully cleaned with chlorhexidine as if for a surgical procedure. A new, sterile, 14 gauge × 5 cm needle should be inserted deep into the swelling. If serum or blood comes out, then it should be withdrawn and the area sprayed with an antibiotic spray. If nothing comes out of the needle, a syringe should be attached and suction should be applied. If nothing comes into the syringe, the needle should be carefully withdrawn. If the syringe fills, with the tip of the needle over a slide, a drop of the contents of the abscess should be carefully expelled. If it is obviously pus the clinician can then

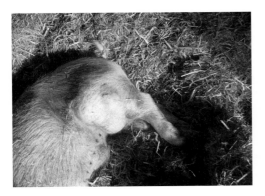

Fig. 12.1. Abscess on stifle.

happily lance the abscess. If required, a smear of the pus can be made and stained appropriately. Haematomata should not be lanced. If pigs are not likely to be slaughtered for human consumption in the near future it is prudent to give a course of antibiotics. If paracentesis reveals an abscess it is essential to provide good drainage. A digital search should be carried out to make sure there is no foreign body. Antibiotics are useful both parenterally and as an aerosol over the incision.

Actinomycosis

The bacterium causing this condition has been renamed *Arcanobacterium pyogenes*. Granulomatous abscesses are commonly seen on the skin but more commonly in individual mammary glands, resulting in a swollen gland and loss of function. Lancing of these abscesses should not be carried out as liquid pus is not forthcoming and often the skin incision fails to heal. The abscesses may also be seen internally at post-mortem. Combinations of penicillin and streptomycin or oxytetracyclines may be tried for treatment, but at best only seem to limit the enlargement of the granulomata. A course of antibiotics can be given when the condition is first seen and repeated if the granulomata burst. If the mammary gland is involved it is prudent to give a prolonged course of antibiotics after farrowing in the hope that further mammary glands will not be affected.

Clostridial cellulitis

Clostridium septicum, Clostridium chauvoei and *Clostridium perfringens* type A have all been isolated from severe cases of cellulitis in pigs. The author suspects that they all start from wounds (normally bite wounds) or injection sites. Penicillin and NSAIDs are the treatment of choice. Many affected animals will survive after the skin has sloughed.

Dermatophilosis

This condition caused by *Dermatophilus congolensis* occurs worldwide but is very rare in pigs compared with other species. It has been recorded as a zoonosis. Crusty lesions will be seen all over the body of adult or growing pigs. The organism will be seen on direct impression smears. Treatment is with parenteral antibiotics and chlorhexidine body washes.

Erysipelas

This is a very common and important disease of pigs. It is caused by *Erysipelothrix rhusiopathiae*, which is ubiquitous in the environment. The disease has zoonotic ramifications in slaughterhouse staff and others closely associated with pigs. It is not primarily a skin disease.

There are four manifestations in pigs.

1. The acute-onset febrile disease in growing pigs, where the fever and inappetence precede the appearance of the classical raised, inflamed, diamond areas on the skin (Fig. 12.2).
2. The subacute form in older pigs which are hardly ill but show the classical diamond-shaped skin lesions.
3. Polyarthritis in growing pigs, which may occur following either of the first two types of infection.
4. The bacteraemia and endocarditis form, which may cause a peracute fatal disease in adult pigs.

The organism is very sensitive to penicillin. This is an excellent treatment in the first two manifestations which show very fast

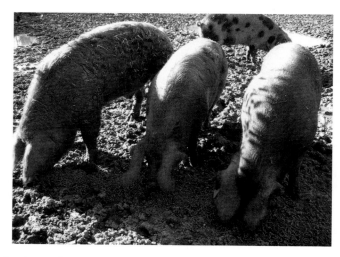

Fig. 12.2. Erysipelas diamonds are difficult to see on coloured pigs.

recovery rates. Pigs showing polyarthritis will recover provided there is no other organism involved. NSAIDs are useful with penicillin to aid recovery.

Once lesions are formed on the heart valves, the pig's days are numbered. High doses of penicillin may bring about a temporary remission. The best treatment is with cephalosporins which have a short slaughter withhold period, so pigs can go for slaughter relatively quickly after treatment.

The vaccine, which can be given to growing pigs and adults, is very effective. One dose followed by a second dose in 4–6 weeks and then every 6 months is the regimen advised.

It should be remembered that *E. rhusiopathiae* will cause abortions.

Greasy pig disease

This is an infectious disease caused by *Staphylococcus hyicus*. It can occur at any age but it occurs mainly in young growing pigs. The piglets may be clinically ill if a large amount of their body surface is affected with the disease. The disease may actually be fatal if piglets are heavily affected. Even with extensive lesions the piglets are not pruritic. The lesions may lead to necrosis of the ear

tips. The organism may be grown in pure culture from swabs taken before treatment. Parenteral antibiotics with topical disinfectant washes are effective treatment. Normally clinicians use amoxicillin with or without clavulinic acid. Dilute chlorohexidine or dilute povidone iodine solutions may be made up into clean plastic dustbins. Piglets may then be totally dipped in the solution before being put on clean shavings and dried under heat lamps.

Porcine dermatitis and nephropathy syndrome

PDNS is a complex condition which is thought to be a hypersensitivity reaction to a severe bacteriological infection. The exact cause is still not known. It is invariably fatal and the clinical manifestation might be confused with CSF, as it is so acute. Affected pigs are severely depressed and totally anorexic. It is normally found in older growing pigs, particularly pigs close to slaughter weight. Mortality rates can be as high as 25% but are normally less. It is extremely rare for the disease to occur in adults. It also might be confused with thrombocytopaenic purpura. The skin lesions are seen over the chest and abdomen together with all four upper legs.

The dermatitis is manifest as large purple lumps. There is no specific test for the disease. On post-mortem the kidneys will be enlarged with a mottled appearance due to multiple small haemorrhages (see Chapter 10). The lymph nodes are also enlarged and haemorrhagic. There is no treatment.

Staphylococcal folliculitis

This is caused by a coagulase-positive *Staphylococcus aureus* and is a distinct clinical entity from greasy pig disease. It can be diagnosed by culture of swabs taken before treatment. It is a disease of growing pigs kept in very dirty conditions. The pigs will show pustules all over their bodies. The condition is self-limiting if the dirty conditions are removed. Antibiotics should not be given as they are unnecessary and will lead to resistant strains of *Staphylococcus* spp.

Streptococcal pustular dermatitis

β-Haemolytic *Streptococcus* spp. can be isolated in pure culture from pustules on the growing pig's skin. It is assumed that they are the cause of the dermatitis. The condition is not self-limiting but does respond very well to single injections of long-acting penicillin.

Ulcerative necrotic granuloma

The cause of these granulomata found on the skin of growing pigs is obscure. *Fusobacterium necrophorum* is often isolated but this is unlikely to be the underlying cause. Treatment with antibiotics needs to be prolonged.

Skin Diseases Caused by Fungi

Ringworm

This is very rare in pigs. It is usually caught from rats or mice and is caused by *Trichophyton mentagrophytes*. Pigs can be infected with *Trichophyton*

verrucosum if they are run with cattle. Treatment in pigs is rarely necessary, as the disease is self-limiting. It should not be confused with pityriasis rosea, which is not caused by a fungus. Ringworm can be diagnosed by seeing fungal hyphae on skin scrapings. Pityriasis rosea will get better in 2 weeks and affect only one or two litters. Ringworm will affect large numbers of pigs and take 4 months to recover. There is no licensed treatment available for pigs in the UK. Griseofulvin should not be used as pigs are a food-producing animal. Enilconazole, licensed for cattle, could be used as a wash under the cascade system. This might be attractive to owners of pet pigs on account of the zoonotic implications with ringworm infections.

Skin Diseases Caused by Parasites

Demodectic mange

This is caused by *Demodex phylloides*. These mites will be found in normal hair follicles. If they occur in very large numbers they will cause small pustular lesions on the body. Normally only when pustules are seen on the face, which when incised will reveal a thick caseous pus containing thousands of mites, is a diagnosis of demodectic mange made. These mites are easily seen without staining under the high power on a microscope. In the author's experience demodectic mange occurs only in animals with a depressed immunity, e.g. animals on prolonged corticosteroid medication or prolonged NSAIDs treatment. Treatment is not easy. Corticosteroid medication and NSAIDs treatment should cease. Antibiotics are helpful. The pigs should be washed at weekly intervals with amitraz solution.

Fleas

Pigs living in close association with humans will be bitten by the human flea *Pulex irritans*. They may also be infested with the cat flea *Ctenocephalides felis*, as well as the sticktight poultry mite *Echidnophaga gallinacea* which is actually a flea. In equatorial Africa they will be infested by the human burrowing flea

Tunga penetrans. Treatment is by dipping or spraying with diazinon.

Flies

There are several species which are attracted to pigs and they can cause physical bite lesions. *Stomoxys calcitrans* will suck blood. Fly strike will occur but it is rare. Both *Lucilia* spp. and *Calliphora* spp. may be involved. Pig muck should be well heaped and kept well away from the pigs. Treatment of fly strike needs to be aggressive with antibiotics, protecting the wound with cream containing acriflavin and BHC, and spraying the pig with diazinon.

Lice

These can be seen with the naked eye as they are large sucking lice called *Haematopinus suis*. They complete their life cycle in a month but they can only be off the pig for 2 days. Therefore the spread of infection is from pig to pig. They cause pruritis. They have been implicated in the spread of pig pox and the blood-borne parasite *Eperythrozoon suis*. Control is accomplished by ivermectin or doramectin treatment. This may be given orally or by injection. If whole herd treatment is carried out for three treatments at 3-weekly intervals, total eradication can easily be achieved.

Sarcoptic mange

This is caused by *Sarcoptes scabiei* var. *suis*. It is the most important and common parasitic disease of pigs (Fig. 12.3). It is a zoonotic disease but human cases resulting from contact with pigs are extremely rare. Crusting particularly on and around the ears and eyes (Fig. 12.4), with pruritis, are the main signs. The mites are readily seen from skin scrapings provided these are not really deep scrapings, as the mites tend to dwell fairly superficially and so a scalpel blade is not required. The author favours the use of a spoon. The preferred site to

sample is the ear margins and inside the pinnae towards the canal. Often the mites can be seen without any preparation just spread on a microscope slide and examined under low power. However many authorities suggest dissolving the crusts in warm 10% w/v potassium hydroxide. This is a fairly lengthy process. The prepatent period can be as short as 10 days but it is normally 2 weeks. The normal picture of an infection is for lesions to be seen a month after new infected pigs are brought on to the premises. If the condition occurs in the ears the self-trauma will result in aural haematomata. Spread of infection occurs via pig-to-pig contact, particularly from the sow to her piglets. Treatment of mange is accomplished with injections of ivermectin or doramectin. Normally a single injection of doramectin will be effective but ivermectin injection should be repeated after 7 days.

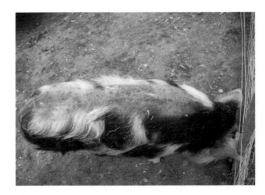

Fig. 12.3. Kunekune pig with sarcoptic mange.

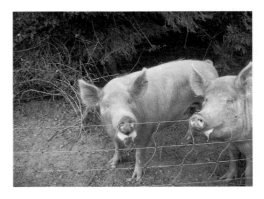

Fig. 12.4. Note the sarcoptic mange around the eyes.

Control should be carried out by 6-monthly oral medication of ivermectins in the food.

Ticks

The species of tick will vary enormously depending on the country. *Ixodes ricinus* will be found on outdoor pigs in the UK. Worldwide, pigs are infested mainly with 'hard ticks' of the family Ixodidae. However in East Africa they may become infested with 'soft ticks' of the genus *Ornithodorus* from the family Argasidae, which spread ASF. *Ornithodorus erraticus* has been implicated in the spread of ASF on the Iberian Peninsula. These ticks are unable to travel more than a metre on their own if not carried by an animal. Therefore to prevent ticks infected with ASF virus from bush pigs infesting domestic pigs, it is important that domestic pigs are double fenced. Ticks can be controlled in the UK with both oral, i.e. in-feed, medication and injections of ivermectin or doramectin. Elsewhere in the world there is a wide range of acaricides available.

Skin Diseases Related to Nutrition

Biotin deficiency

The main signs are hair loss and hoof lesions. Normally hoof lesions precede skin lesions. Treatment with biotin in the food readily controls the condition and can be used as a diagnostic tool.

Iodine deficiency

This is an extremely rare condition of piglets born to iodine-deficient sows. The piglets will be hairless but will not show goitre.

Parakeratosis

This is caused by a deficiency of zinc in the diet or by a conditioned deficiency from high levels of phytic acid in soy. It is found in young growing pigs and is manifest as scaly papules. Diagnosis should be made with a skin biopsy as testing the blood for zinc levels is unreliable. Treatment is restoring the zinc level in the diet to 100 ppm taking account of the level of soy in the food. The response to treatment can be used as a diagnostic tool.

Vitamin A deficiency

This is extremely rare and is manifest as a generalized seborrhoea. It is seen in weak piglets born to deficient sows. Other signs of vitamin A deficiency, e.g. neurological signs, are going to be much more obvious than the skin disease.

Vitamin B deficiency

Other than biotin deficiency which is relatively common, niacin, pantothenic acid and riboflavin deficiencies have been reported as well but they are extremely rare. Skin disease signs are very variable but are usually seen as dry scaly areas. Total resorption will occur if the diet is corrected.

Skin Diseases due to Miscellaneous Causes

Aural haematoma

These are normally caused by violent head shaking caused by pruritic parasitic conditions. Normally the swelling is on the median aspect of the ear between the cartilage and the skin. The condition is usually restricted to lop-eared animals. The underlying cause must be treated, i.e. a doramectin injection to kill the mange mites, and if the swollen ear is left it will result in permanent scarring called a 'cauliflower ear'. On no account should practitioners lance these swellings as they will result in severe haemorrhage. They may be drained with a sterile needle and syringe and then filled with a long-acting corticosteroid. However this is rarely success-ful in the author's experience. In theory in a pet pig the haematoma could be drained under a GA and then buttons could be sutured both inside and outside the ear in a similar manner to a dog with an aural haematoma, but this is outside the author's experience.

Bite wounds

These are common after pig groups have been mixed and they may be severe. They require aggressive antibiotic treatment. They should not be sutured but allowed to heal by secondary intention. Precautions should be taken to avoid fly strike. Oxytetracycline aerosols are useful.

Burns

These sadly are common (see Chapter 7).

Callus

These are formed on adult pigs over bony prominences when the pigs are bedded down on concrete. Rapid provision of soft surfaces is vital or ulcers will be formed. If ulcers have formed the animal should be given antibiotics and NSAIDs and the ulcers should be treated with oily creams. A similar condition will be seen on the carpi of baby piglets made to suckle on hard concrete.

Frostbite

This will involve the extremities of outdoor pigs in severe weather conditions. It is a very painful condition. NSAIDs are helpful.

Melanomas

These are extremely rare and in the author's experience occur only on the flanks of black pigs. Diagnosis is not a problem and so

there is little need for a biopsy. Excision is unlikely to be required.

Juvenile papillomas

The cause for these is obscure but they are likely to be of viral origin. They will occur in unweaned piglets and regress spontaneously. Diagnosis will be made on clinical signs. No treatment is required. Often just one or two litters are affected and then no further cases are seen.

Pemphigus

Autoimmune diseases are seen in pigs but they are extremely rare. Diagnosis will be achieved by ruling out other causes for the erythematous, pruritic patches on the skin. Diagnosis could be confirmed by histopath-ology. Treatment is with corticosteroids in pet pigs. Initially dexamethazone can be injected at 2 mg/25 kg every 48 h with antibiotic cover. Then when the inflammation and infection has decreased, oral medication can be continued with prednisolone at 1 mg/kg and oral doxycycline at 20 mg/kg. Treatment is far from satisfactory as the condition will recur, particularly in the warm months of the year. Oily creams are helpful. Euthanasia is probably indicated in the long term.

Porcine ulcerative dermatitis syndrome

This rare condition resembles healing of widespread burns and tends to regress spon-taneously. The cause is unknown. It is likely to be viral. The treatment is soft clean bed-ding and oily creams.

Pressure sores

These are commonly seen in overweight adult pigs kept on concrete. Their occurrence is minimal now that pigs are no longer kept in crates. Antibiotic injections and sprays are helpful. It is vital to address the cause of the problem. Pigs should be supplied with soft clean bedding.

Recurrent dermatosis

This is a condition of sows which tends to recur each time they come into the farrowing house. The cause is unknown. The signs are large round areas of roughened skin which is non-pruritic or painful. There is no treatment.

Sunburn

This is possible in outdoor white pigs in the UK. It is seen much more commonly in the tropics if there is no shade or mud wallows. It is not likely in black pigs and has not been recorded in Saddlebacks or Kunekune pigs. The author has never seen the condition in Vietnamese pigs either in the UK or the Far East. The pigs most at risk are white sows in a group with a black boar or a white boar with a group of black sows. Pigs should be brought into the shade and be cooled with water. Severely affected animals should be given antibiotics and NSAIDs. Lesions should be treated with oily creams. Fly control is important otherwise the lesions will not heal.

Uticaria

This is rare in pigs and is called 'hives'. In theory it could be caused by a contact allergy or even a food allergy but these are unlikely. The likely cause is an allergic reaction to an insect bite, usually a biting fly or a tick. The whole of the pig's body will be covered in raised plaques. This is a peracute condition. The pig's temperature will be raised. The respiratory rate may be raised. The condition is normally self-limiting within a few hours. Cooling the pig with cold water from a hose is helpful. Severe reactions can be treated with systemic corticosteroids, e.g. dexamethazone by injection.

Non-infectious Skin Diseases of Neonatal Piglets

Aplasia cutis

This condition is extremely rare and is likely to be a simple autosomal recessive trait. It is seen in several breeds of pig and is found worldwide. It is manifest as a single round area of the body totally lacking any skin, which rapidly turns to an ulcer. Clinicians must be mindful of welfare as in the author's experience the lesion is not like a normal ulcer and does not seem to heal. The piglet may grow so that the lesion will appear to be smaller. This is relative and each case needs careful assessment. Euthanasia is likely to be the most humane procedure.

Bite wounds on the faces of neonatal piglets

These may be seen as early as 24 h as piglets fight to retain their nipple. Removing the canines soon after birth with a pair of nail clippers may help to prevent the condition. In the majority of cases the wounds heal very rapidly unless they become infected with *S. hyicus* and the piglets develop greasy pig disease.

Cutaneous asthenia

This may be an inherited condition as it is restricted to Saddleback and Large White pigs. The skin is hyper-elastic and can be raised up in folds without the piglet showing pain. Normally there are no other problems and the pigs can be reared through to slaughter. Obviously the pigs should not be kept for breeding.

Dermatosis vegetans

This is a rare congenital inherited condition of pigs, seen in Landrace pigs. The coronary band does not develop normally so that at birth the feet are not normal. The piglets should be destroyed and the breeding of the sire and dam should be investigated.

Epitheliogenesis imperfecta

This is a rare congenital condition which is inherited. It is also called aplasia cutis (see above).

Inherited congenital goitre

This very rare congenital condition is seen in Landrace and Large White pigs. It is thought to be autosomal recessive. The piglets are totally hairless. Hairlessness is also shown in Mexican pigs but these do not have goitre. They can often be reared as normal for slaughter. None of the litter should be kept for breeding. The genetics of the sire and dam should be checked.

Pityriasis rosea

This is an inherited condition which appears in young suckling pigs. It is self-limiting. This is the reason why it is so common, as often the affected piglets are kept in error for breeding. It is manifest as large, round, red scabby plaques. These are not pruritic. It has no links with any fungal condition. No treatment is required.

Pressure sores

These will be seen within 24 h of birth on the knees of piglets raised on very rough concrete. The source of the problem should be removed and the piglets treated with oily creams. It should be stressed that this is a welfare issue.

Thrombocytopaenic purpura

This is an isoimmune condition affecting young suckling pigs. The affected pigs show large cyanotic areas. They also have multiple haemorrhages. Normally the whole litter starts to die 48 h after ingesting the colostrum. Sometimes smaller pigs which have not had much colostrum will survive. The condition can only occur in sows, not in first litter gilts.

On post-mortem the whole carcass will show multiple haemorrhages in all muscles including the myocardium. Also, all of the lymph nodes will be engorged with blood. There is normally no evidence of jaundice. Obviously the piglets are very shocked and warmth is required. Fluid replacer with multivitamins and antibiotics should be offered. Piglets should not be injected as they will haemorrhage at the injection site. Vitamin K does not seem to be helpful. To prevent the condition the same sire should not be used again on that sow.

13 Multisystemic Diseases

African Swine Fever

This highly contagious disease with a high mortality is caused by an iridovirus. It is a totally different virus from that causing CSF. Clinically it is impossible to differentiate the two diseases. It is found mainly in Africa but there have been outbreaks in Southern European countries. It occurs in Central Asia. It also occurs in the Caribbean and South America. It is a notifiable disease in the UK. It affects domestic pigs and wild boar. It does not cause clinical signs but occurs in bush pigs (*Potamochoerus porcus*) and warthogs (*Phacochoerus aethiopicus*). Both these species of pig are carriers and spread the disease to domestic pigs. The disease can be spread by pig lice and soft ticks. The virus will survive for long periods of time in meat products. The severity of the clinical signs is extremely variable but in the majority of outbreaks they are acute after an incubation period of 5–7 days. Affected pigs will have a high rectal temperature and be hyperaemic. They will be anorexic, depressed and recumbent. They often vomit and show respiratory distress. There may be epistaxis and bloody diarrhoea. Death will follow in 48 h. The severe disease may result in neurological signs. If the less severe signs occur there is a lower viraemia and pigs will recover. There may be some transient joint inflammation. The first manifestation may be abortions. Diagnosis in live pigs is made by PCR and a variety of methods have been described. Virus isolation and diagnosis can also be carried out by replication of virus in primary macrophages and detection of infected cells by the characteristic haemadsorption of red blood cells around infected cells (Coggins, 1968). Diagnosis can be made by serum ELISA but this has a reduced sensitivity compared with PCR. At post-mortem the spleen, tonsils and gastro-hepatic lymph nodes should be submitted for virus isolation. This can be verified on PCR. There are petechiae in the kidneys, lymph nodes and heart.

Strict import controls on pigs, pig products and pig by-products should prevent the spread of this disease. However, illegal imports, accidentally or intentionally, continue to cause this disease to spread. The ban on swill feeding reduces the risk of exposure of pigs to illegally imported infected meat products. However, accidental exposure, particularly in farms with outdoor pigs and pet pigs, remains a risk. The infection of wild boar from exposure to infected meat is also possible, which could increase the risk of spread to domestic pigs if they come in contact with wild boar. Wild boar constitute a risk of trans-boundary spread in areas where wild boar are common.

There is no treatment or vaccine available. However the prospects for vaccine development are good.

Anthrax

This rapidly fatal disease in cattle is not nearly so acute in pigs, although of course it is still a zoonosis and is notifiable in the UK and throughout the world. It is extremely rare in the UK and most other temperate countries; however it is seen more often in tropical countries. The disease is caused by *Bacillus anthracis*. While the organism is in the pig it may multiply and is sensitive to penicillin. If the blood or other body fluids are allowed to leak out of the pig into the fresh air, the bacteria will form spores which are very resistant to boiling and most disinfectants. These spores can survive in the soil for decades. It is therefore vital that infected pigs are either burnt or buried in quicklime. Pigs can develop three forms: the enteric form, the septicaemic form and the skin form. Pigs can become infected with the enteric form in various ways: ingesting the spores in the soil when rooting, from biting flies and most importantly from eating contaminated foodstuffs. Pigs can develop the septicaemic form as a result of the enteric form. The organism normally gets into the circulation via the tonsils. Pigs can also become infected with the skin form through contamination of wounds. The septicaemic form is rare in pigs. The most common manifestation is swelling of the throat with difficulty in breathing. Pigs will have a raised rectal temperature and will be depressed and anorexic. Mortality is under 20%. However, recovery will be slow and often areas of skin become necrotic and slough off. Diagnosis can be carried out by seeing the organism with its tell-tale capsule in smears taken from subcutaneous oedema of the throat and stained with MacFadean's stain. Smears should be taken on to blood slides and air-dried. These should then be fixed by heat from a naked flame. Old methylene blue should be applied to the slide when cool and left for 30 s. It should be washed off with running water. Once the slide is dry it can be examined under oil emersion. The rectangular bacteria in chains will take up the stain and the capsule will be clearly seen as a translucent covering.

It must be remembered that anthrax is a zoonotic disease and therefore the wisdom of treating pigs with anthrax is in question. Certainly the meat from infected pigs should not be used for human consumption.

There is a vaccine available in certain countries but it is not licensed for use in the UK or elsewhere in the EU.

Classical Swine Fever

The disease is also called hog cholera in the USA. It is caused by a pestivirus. It is a highly contagious disease and cannot clinically be differentiated from ASF. It is found worldwide but the UK, Australia, New Zealand and the USA are free of the disease. On the whole, Europe is free but there are sporadic outbreaks. It is a notifiable disease in the UK. It affects domestic pigs and wild boar may harbour the virus, but the main transmission is from pig to pig. Like ASF the virus may be spread by feeding pig products to pigs. The CSF virus is more fragile than the ASF virus and is readily killed by heat. Historically this resulted in the boiling of swill, but now swill feeding is banned in most countries. The normal manifestation of the disease is the severe acute form. However, the chronic form is also seen. Pigs die eventually within a couple of months. The normal incubation period is 3–7 days with death in 10 days. Affected pigs will have a high fever and constipation which is then followed by diarrhoea. There are haemorrhages and cyanotic areas on the skin, particularly on the legs. There are often neurological signs which are not just from the high fever. There may be abortions. The disease can be suspected on clinical grounds. Whole blood in ethylene diamine tetra-acetic acid (EDTA) (normally a purple-topped tube) can be taken for virus isolation. Clotted samples (normally a red-topped tube) are useful for serology. On post-mortem there are widespread haemorrhages and ecchymoses found in the lymph nodes, spleen, bladder and larynx. The pathognomic sign is the ecchymotic kidneys, the so-called 'turkey egg' kidneys. There is a non-suppurative encephalitis. Antigen detection can be carried out using direct immunofluorescence on frozen sections of the tonsil. RT-PCR can be used to differentiate CSF virus from other pestiviruses. There is no treatment and most countries adopt a slaughter policy. In countries where the disease is endemic there is a vaccine which may be used. If wild boar are involved there is a live vaccine, which can be put in bait to attempt to control the disease.

Clostridium novyi Infection

This bacterium used to be called *Clostridium oedematiens*. It is type B *Clostridium novyi* which normally affects pigs. It is possible that type A will also cause a similar condition. It occurs worldwide. It causes sudden death in adult pigs and large fat pigs because it produces a powerful toxin. It replicates only in an anaerobic situation. This occurs in the liver of a pig affected with chronic pneumonia or severe enteritis. On post-mortem the liver is full of gas and looks like foam rubber. Diagnosis can be confirmed on FAT or PCR on the liver tissue. Post-mortem changes occur extremely rapidly, so trying to confirm the diagnosis by seeing the organism on smears is unreliable.

There is no treatment as the animals will be found dead. However, controlling the predisposing conditions such as the pneumonia or enteritis with antibiotics might be helpful. There is no licensed vaccine for pigs in the UK. Sheep vaccine can be used on the cascade system and seems to be effective.

Foot and Mouth Disease

FMD is a highly contagious disease which occurs as an acute disease in pigs. It is caused by an aphthovirus. It is notifiable throughout the world. It is not found in the UK and mainland Europe except occasionally there may be incursions from the East. It is not found in the USA, Australia or New Zealand. It is found in Asia, Africa and South America.

There are seven different serotypes. 'A', 'O' and 'C' are classically described as European serotypes. They are the only serotypes which have been found in Europe. They are also found in Asia and Africa. The Asia serotype is restricted to Asia. The three South African serotypes, 'SAT 1', 'SAT 2' and 'SAT 3', are found in Africa and on occasions have been found in Asia.

The virus is extremely contagious and can infect pigs by inhalation, ingestion and by skin wounds. The most important for an initial infection is when pigs eat an infected piece of meat. However, when an outbreak has become established then the respiratory route becomes extremely important. There is a massive outpouring of virus in exhaled air. With housed pigs kept in modern pig houses with good ventilation, there is a 'plume' effect. This can spread the virus over wide areas.

Clinical signs are seen in all ages of pig. They are very marked and unlikely to be missed by observant practitioners. There will be a sudden onset of severe lameness in the whole herd. Piglets and growing pigs will actually squeal if made to move. All ages will have hunched backs and be reluctant to move. They should have their feet washed with water, ideally from a hose, to clean off any debris and then the small raised areas will be seen. These rapidly turn into vesicles approximately 1 cm in diameter. Vesicles will be seen on the tongue and the snout, which make the pig produce excessive saliva. Disinfectants should not be used to clean the feet as they will lessen the chances of virus isolation.

Leptospirosis

This can be considered to be a multisystemic disease as it can cause meningitis, jaundice and fever in young pigs. However its main manifestation occurs in the reproductive system of sows which leads to abortions and stillbirths.

Malignant Catarrhal Fever

Malignant catarrhal fever (MCF), a cattle disease which is caused by ovine herpes virus type 2 (Ov-HV2), has been recorded in pigs. The main clinical signs are: corneal opacity, ocular discharge and respiratory distress. Diagnosis is made by PCR. The disease is contracted from sheep.

Porcine Dermatitis and Nephropathy Syndrome

PDNS is normally a disease of large fattening pigs. It often occurs at the same time as PMWS. There is no direct link between the two diseases. Some authorities suggest that there is a link between PDNS and *Pasteurella multocida*. The syndrome is likely to be a hypersensitivity reaction to either a virus or a bacterium. Affected animals have confusing clinical signs. The pigs are normally pyrexic. The most obvious other sign is the marked, purplish, widespread skin coloration. This is mainly on the hindquarters. There is no treatment and euthanasia is advised. On postmortem there is general lymphadenopathy with the kidneys swollen and petichiated. There is also pneumonia.

Porcine Reproductive and Respiratory Syndrome

PRRS is a disease which affects all ages of pig when there is no immunity in the herd. This situation is now rare as not only is the virus widespread but also there are many good vaccines available. Sows will show respiratory distress but not marked pyrexia. Only a few animals will show the classical sign of blue ears. Abortions will occur and as time goes on there will be a larger percentage of stillbirths and returns to service. There will be a sharp rise in the number of weak piglets born. These will have conjunctivitis. Many will not survive. The number of deaths in the weaner pens will rise. The pigs will have pneumonia. Post-mortems will not be very helpful as there will be a rise in the number of other conditions usually seen in the herd. Frozen tonsil samples will reveal the virus. Antibiotics will not be effective in controlling the disease. Vaccination is the key.

Post-weaning Multisystemic Wasting Syndrome

This disease is caused by PCV-2 and so PMWS is often called porcine circovirus. The infection is very widespread in the UK and throughout the world with the exception of Australia and New Zealand. It was first reported in Canada in 1996 (Fig. 13.1).

The virus spreads oro-nasally with an incubation period of 10–14 days. Piglets can also become infected in the womb. Passive immunity protects against clinical disease but not against infection. Presence of the virus predisposes to infections of PDNS. The presence of torque teno virus (TTV), which is a ubiquitous and species-specific virus that infects domestic pigs and wild boar, can serve as a 'trigger' or

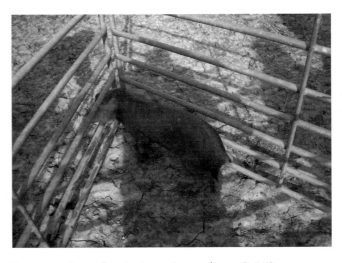

Fig. 13.1. A pig with post-weaning multisystemic wasting syndrome (PMWS).

co-factor for PCV-2 in the pathogenesis of PMWS (Novosel *et al.*, 2012). Infection in a herd will increase pre-weaning mortality but signs are not seen until after weaning particularly in 7- to 9-week-old growing pigs. As the name suggests, there are several systems affected and therefore there are a large number of clinical signs, namely: wasting, pallor, pyrexia, rough coat, jaundice, lymphadenopathy, diarrhoea and death (Fig. 13.1). Mortality in totally naive herds may be two-thirds of the pigs. The non-affected pigs will appear to be totally normal. As there is no treatment and no chance of recovery after the development of clinical signs, affected animals should be destroyed as soon as possible. Fattening pigs and adults are not affected. Abortions and stillbirths will be seen but these signs are not common.

PME will reveal a pale, often jaundiced, generally wasted carcass with all of the lymph nodes swollen, firm and pale. The lungs fail to collapse. The liver will be small and will often have white foci. The kidneys may be normal but more commonly they are pale and also have white foci. There are ulcers in the stomach. The intestines are distended with watery contents. There may be a typhlitis. Histopathological samples of the foci in the liver and kidneys are helpful with diagnosis. Histopathological samples of enlarged lymph nodes and the tonsil will show basophilic inclusion bodies. Bacteriology is not helpful as there is often a wide range of secondary bacteria. Diagnosis can be made on these post-mortem signs together with PCR. The presence of antibodies in aborted fetal fluids is diagnostic.

Control is by attention to strict hygiene and movement restriction. The virus is spread around the farm by pig-to-pig contact. This can also be indirect by a needle, surgical instrument, muck or people. Stressed animals are far more likely to become diseased. Vaccination of growing pigs against PCV-2 has been shown to be highly effective in decreasing the prevalence and severity of porcine circovirus-associated disease (O'Neill *et al.*, 2012). Studies have shown that a substantial number of piglets are born viraemic and appear to be healthy. The consequences of early, subclinical PCV-2 infection of pigs are largely unknown but it seems logical to assume that reduction or elimination of vertical PCV-2 transmission is beneficial. One way to reduce dam viraemia and infection of piglets may be through dam vaccination. This was shown be effective (O'Neill *et al.*, 2012). Vaccination of piglets before weaning is definitely helpful.

Swine Erysipelas

Erysipelas in pigs is caused by the bacterium *Erysipelothrix rhusiopathiae* (formerly *Erysipelothrix insidiosa*) that is found widely in wild birds and rodents. The organism is capable of survival in a damp environment (including soil) for up to 6 months. Thus exposure of pigs to any of these sources has the potential to lead to disease if the animals are not immune. Many strains exist but two predominate in cases of pig disease.

Erysipelas is a true multisystemic disease. It can affect the circulatory system in two ways. It can be a peracute disease with a septicaemia. This may be so peracute that the pig is found dead with blue discoloration of the skin and the extremities, together with petechiae throughout the carcass. It can also cause endocarditis in adults. This may also result in sudden death. If endocarditis is suspected the pig should be given prolonged high doses of penicillin and this against expectations may resolve the condition.

The most common form of erysipelas is the acute form which is mainly seen in growing pigs rather than in adults. Pigs will be lethargic and off their food. Rectal temperatures will rise to over 42°C. The classic diamond-shaped, raised red lesions will appear. The red colour will not be seen in black pigs but the lesions will still be felt on the skin. As the disease is very sensitive to treatment with penicillin the mortality is very low, but without treatment it can be up to 20%. In most cases the skin lesions will regress as the rectal temperature falls and the appetite of the pig returns. In some cases the skin lesions, because of secondary infections with *Staphylococcus* spp., will become necrotic and there will be a sloughing of the skin. In these cases the pig will take weeks to regain health and start putting on weight.

The high fever experienced by gilts suffering from this acute form of erysipelas will lead to abortions if they are in the later stages of pregnancy. This is just because of the pyrexia. With treatment not only should the animals receive penicillin but also NSAIDs to reduce the fever. Practitioners should warn pig keepers of this possible sequel to the disease. However, erysipelas will cause abortions per se. The organism can readily be cultured from aborted fetuses and afterbirths. Ten days after the abortion, serum from affected pigs will show high titres against erysipelas. This is an even more significant finding if the titre is low on the day of the abortion. If sows and gilts suffer from erysipelas early in pregnancy there will be high levels of returns to service. If they are infected at 2–3 months of pregnancy they will go to term but produce mummified piglets.

Erysipelas will also cause arthritis in growing pigs and replacement gilts. This is thought to be immune mediated and often is seen in pigs which have not shown the clinical signs, although normally their pen mates have experienced the disease. In the author's experience the condition is incurable, even with aggressive antibiotic and NSAID treatment, and therefore euthanasia must be recommended.

Vaccination is inexpensive and should be recommended for all classes of pig, both commercial and on smallholdings. It should be recommended for both growing pigs and adults. The vaccine is normally an inactivated vaccine in an aqueous adjuvant, which should be injected im. Pigs need to be a minimum of 6 weeks of age before the first injection. The second injection should be given approximately 4 weeks after the first injection. Then the cover needs to be kept up by 6-monthly boosters. Sows and gilts can be injected during pregnancy but if possible this should not be in the two final weeks. Immune sows will give passive immunity to their piglets for up to 9 weeks, so vaccination between 6 and 9 weeks will give continuous protection.

Other methods of control include removing sources of contamination. This is difficult in outside pigs but is worthwhile as the control measures are useful for other diseases. As wild birds are a source of contamination they should be kept away from pigs and particularly away from pig feed. Poultry, particularly turkeys, are a source of contamination and should be kept separate. Rodent control is important. Faecal hygiene should be improved with empty and clean scrape-through systems. The equivalent measure in outdoor pigs is moving to fresh ground. This will be helpful in controlling erysipelas. Some authors consider sheep to be a risk to pigs. However, in the author's experience it is the pig which is a danger to the sheep. When ewes are lambing down in the same accommodation as pigs there is an increase in the number of cases of joint ill in lambs. *E. rhusiopathiae* can be isolated from inflamed joints.

In acute outbreaks of erysipelas in growing pigs the recommended preventive treatment is amoxicillin in the water. This should only be used as an emergency treatment while vaccination is being carried out.

Swine Vesicular Disease

The importance of this disease, which is caused by an enterovirus, is that it is indistinguishable clinically from FMD. It was first observed in Italy in 1966 but was not seen in the UK until 1972. It occurred sporadically in the UK until the early 1980s. It was last seen in Europe in Italy in 2005. It has been seen in the Far East but not in Africa, the New World, Australia or New Zealand.

The virus can penetrate intact skin particularly on the coronary band. It can also gain entry via the gut. It tracts through the lymph system and rapidly causes a viraemia. It will cause mild pyrexia within 2 days. Lameness through pain in the feet is the most prominent sign. Animals are reluctant to move. Unlike FMD, it does not occur in ruminants. Vesicles may be seen on the tongue and snout but foot lesions are the most noticeable. The incubation period is 2 days but can be as long as a week. It is spread mainly by pig-to-pig contact. The virus can survive in faeces for several months. Swill feeding, which is now banned in the UK, is often the cause of an outbreak.

Diagnosis can be made with RT-PCR which will distinguish the virus from FMD. At the present time there would be a slaughter policy if the virus was located in the UK.

14 Notifiable Diseases

The World Organization for Animal Health is also known as the Office International des Epizooties (OIE). This organization monitors specific epizootic diseases agreed by the member governments. Each member government has its own particular list of diseases. In the UK the list is compiled by DEFRA. This chapter concentrates on the notifiable diseases which occur in pigs, whether just in pigs or in other species as well as in pigs. Certain diseases occur in several species and others are only found in single species.

FMD and rabies are two main notifiable diseases of pigs and other species in the UK, with a high media concern. They are shown in Table 14.1. It is vital that practitioners who are attending any pig farm, whether large or small, are vigilant for FMD. It is extremely likely that the next outbreak of FMD in the UK will come from pigs via inappropriate feeding of foreign pig products to pigs by mistake. Swill feeding is banned in the UK. In other countries where FMD is exotic it is just as important that practitioners are vigilant, particularly if swill feeding is practised. The author feels that the keeping of pet pigs is a particular danger worldwide. Biosecurity is obviously harder with outdoor pigs. Birds could easily spread disease (Fig. 14.1).

Rabies is a fatal zoonotic disease. It is possible that pigs can become infected from the bite of a carnivore, another pig or a bat, but it is very unlikely that the first case of rabies will occur in a pig in any country free of rabies.

Table 14.2 shows further diseases monitored by DEFRA in the UK and Table 14.3 shows further diseases monitored by the OIE worldwide.

Disease patterns are changing constantly and practitioners are advised to consult their national regulatory authority.

African Swine Fever

ASF was first recognized in Kenya in 1921 by R.E. Montgomery. He recognized the disease as an acute haemorrhagic fever infecting domestic pigs of European origin. They became infected from the symptomless carrier, the warthog *Phacochocerus africanus* (Fig. 14.2). It was soon realized that the soft tick of the Argasidae family was also a reservoir of the virus and was a vector. The virus could also be found in the bush pig, *Potamochoerus larvatus*, and the giant forest hog, *Hylochoerus meinertzhagani*. Double fences are required to protect domestic pigs from picking up infected soft ticks from wild pigs (Fig. 14.3).

ASF first was recorded in Europe in Portugal in 1957. It occurred through swill

Table 14.1. The two main notifiable diseases of pigs and other farm livestock in the UK.

Disease	Species affected	Disease type	Occurred last in UK
Foot and mouth disease (FMD)	Pigs, ruminants and SACs	Exotic	2007
Rabies	Pigs and all mammals	Exotic and zoonotic	1970

SAC, South American camelid.

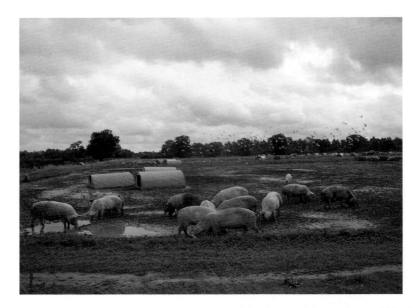

Fig. 14.1. Outdoor pigs make biosecurity difficult because of the danger of disease from wild birds.

Table 14.2. Six further notifiable diseases of pigs alone or pigs and other farm livestock in the UK.

Disease	Species affected	Disease type	Occurred last in UK
African swine fever (ASF)	Pigs	Exotic	Never
Anthrax	Ruminants, pigs and SACs	Zoonotic	2006
Aujeszky's disease	Pigs	Exotic	1989
Classical swine fever (CSF)	Pigs	Exotic	2000
Swine vesicular disease (SVD)	Pigs	Exotic	1982
Vesicular stomatitis	Cattle and pigs	Exotic	Never

feeding. It spread rapidly throughout the Iberian Peninsula and took over 30 years to eradicate. Other countries like France, Italy, Belgium and the Netherlands have had outbreaks but, except in Sardinia, it has never become endemic in Europe and the disease has managed to be eradicated. It has crossed the Atlantic to the Caribbean and Brazil, but has also managed to be eradicated in these areas.

At the time of writing the disease is reported in most sub-Saharan countries in Africa including Madagascar. Elsewhere it is restricted to Russia, Armenia and Sardinia.

Table 14.3. Further diseases affecting pigs, either pigs alone or pigs and other farm livestock, being monitored by the Office International des Epizooties worldwide.

Disease	Species affected	Disease type	Occurred last in UK
Japanese encephalitis	Pigs	Exotic and zoonotic	Never
Leptospirosis	Cattle, sheep, goats, pigs and SACs	Endemic and zoonotic	Present
Nipah virus encephalitis	Pigs	Exotic and zoonotic	Never
Old world screw-worm	Cattle, sheep, goats, pigs and SACs	Exotic	Never
Porcine cysticercosis	Pigs	Rare and zoonotic	Present
Porcine reproductive and respiratory syndrome (PRRS)	Pigs	Endemic	Present
Teschen/Talfan disease	Pigs	Rare in Eastern Europe	Never
Transmissible gastroenteritis (TGE)	Pigs	Very rare	Present
Trichinellosis	Pigs	Exotic and zoonotic	Never
Tularaemia	Sheep and pigs	Exotic and zoonotic	Never

SAC, South American camelid.

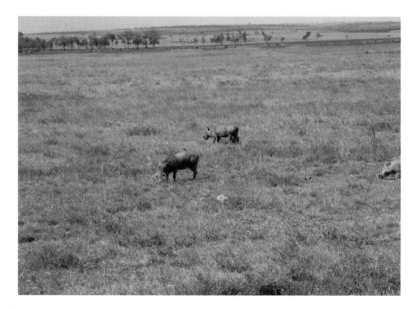

Fig. 14.2. Warthogs in Africa can spread disease.

It has never occurred in the UK but clinicians should always be vigilant. In Russia it is found as far north as St Petersburg and Murmansk. In these northern areas it is spread in a domestic pig cycle. In sub-Saharan Africa it is spread mainly in a wildlife cycle. Molecular epidemiological research has greatly improved our understanding of the two different modes of spread of the disease.

Aujeszky's Disease

This virus disease was endemic in pig populations almost worldwide. It is found in rodents, which spread the disease. It has very rarely been reported in cattle, sheep and man. It has been eradicated from the UK, most of Europe and most of North America. It has never been seen in North Africa or Australia.

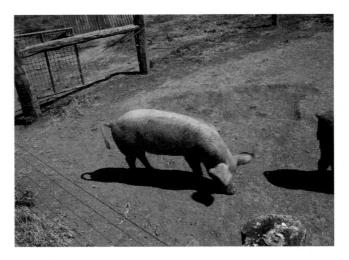

Fig. 14.3. Pigs need extra double fencing in Southern Africa.

Classical Swine Fever

This solely pig disease is a totally separate disease from ASF. It is also called hog cholera. It has been eradicated from the UK and large areas of Europe and North America, by the use of vaccination in the 1960s. It still occurs in other areas of the world and has the ability to cause serious pandemics, so clinicians must be constantly vigilant and aware of the danger of the disease which could be spread by pig products.

Foot and Mouth Disease

At the time of writing, the main hotspots for FMD are North Africa and the Middle East. The main strains are 'SAT 2', 'O' and 'A'. Pigs are not prominent in these areas on account of religious beliefs and therefore the disease has not been reported in pigs. The main reports in pigs have been in Taiwan, which is experiencing the isolation of an 'O' strain found on routine serological surveillance.

Japanese Encephalitis

This disease is also called Japanese B encephalitis. It is caused by a flavivirus. It occurs in pigs, horses and man. Wild birds are the reservoir host. It is spread by mosquitoes. The pig is the build-up host for horses and man. The main sign in pigs is abortion. In man there is fever and severe headache leading to encephalitis. The mortality can be as high as 30%. The virus is restricted to Asia, mainly on Pacific Islands from Japan to the Philippines. The American state of Hawaii is the only part of the USA at risk. There is a good vaccine for pigs. This should be used to limit the danger to man.

Leptospirosis

This disease is not notifiable in the UK and in fact it is not that uncommon. However, it is of interest worldwide because of its zoonotic implications. It causes mummified pigs, abortions and stillbirths. It can on rare occasions cause illness in young pigs. Serological evidence of the infection is widespread in the UK and in the rest of the world. The main serovars are *Leptospira pomona*, *L. bratislava*, *L. grippotyphosa*, *L. icterohaemorrhagiae* and *L. canicola*.

Nipah Virus Encephalitis

This is caused by a paramyovirus. It was first found in Malaysia in 1998. It is a zoonotic disease which causes encephalitis in humans and pigs. The wild reservoir for the virus is in fruit bats of the genus *Pteropus*. The virus is closely related to the Hendra virus. More recently in outbreaks of Nipah virus in India and Bangladesh, pigs do not appear to be involved and humans have contracted the disease directly from fruit bats.

In outbreaks in intensive pig units there is a rapid spread of the disease which can cause up to 40% mortality. Encephalitis is seen in the adults. Growing pigs have a fever and a marked cough, which is why it is called the 'barking pig syndrome'. Diagnosis can be made with a PCR. There is no treatment available for pigs. Euthanasia should be carried out immediately not only on welfare grounds but also to limit the spread of the disease. There is no vaccine available. Humans working with pigs are most at risk of contracting the disease.

Old World Screw-worm

This is *Chysomyia bezziana*, an obligatory wound parasite. It does not develop in carcasses or decomposing organic matter. It is found in Africa, India and South-east Asia. In pigs and humans it produces a particularly unpleasant myiasis. It will affect other mammals. The adult fly has a dark metallic-green body and is rarely seen. It can lay up to 500 eggs around a wound or in even a natural orifice contaminated with blood or mucus. The mature third-stage larvae develop within a week. They are nearly 2 cm long and quickly burrow into the skin. In untreated wounds the destructive effect of the maggots may kill the pig within a few hours.

Affected pigs should receive an injection of 200 µg ivermectin/kg to kill the maggots. They should also receive antibiotics to combat the secondary infection and dexamethazone to limit the shock. The wound should be dressed with a cream containing acriflavin and BHC.

Samples of the maggots should be preserved and sent off to the official veterinary headquarters so that appropriate measures to control the fly can be undertaken.

Porcine Cysticercosis

This is caused by the larval form of the tapeworm *Taenia solium*, which is found in the small intestine of humans. The larval form or metacestode is a fluid-filled bladder-like structure found in the musculature of pigs. The real danger to man is ingestion of the eggs which then become metacestodes in the musculature of man. They may also form in the brain or ocular tissue with disastrous results. The adult worms can relatively easily be eliminated from humans with anthelmintics. The metacestodes in pig meat can be killed by prolonged freezing or by aggressive cooking.

Porcine Reproductive and Respiratory Syndrome

This disease is widespread in most pig-producing countries, including the UK. It is not seen in Australia or New Zealand. It is caused by an arterivirus. Sequence and antigenic analysis suggests that the European strain is different from the New World strain. The disease is monitored by the OIE. Further information on this syndrome can be seen in Chapter 13.

Rabies

From a notifiable standpoint this disease is much more important in other species. However, it does occur in the pig, and so in Asia and Africa veterinarians need to remember this disease as a differential for other neurological conditions.

Swine Vesicular Disease

The importance of this viral disease of pigs is its similarity clinically to FMD. It is rarely reported worldwide. It was reported in two separate outbreaks in Italy in 2012. Whether it is under-reported or whether it is a rare disease is difficult to establish.

It is caused by an enterovirus. It was first recorded in Italy in 1966 and in the UK in 1972.

It is a more robust virus than that causing FMD. The normal route of infection is oral. It has an incubation period as short as 48 h. Clinically it is exactly the same as FMD with fever and lameness being the most prominent signs. In very rare cases there are neurological signs.

Historically the outbreaks have been linked to swill feeding, so it is hoped the virus will not return to the UK as swill feeding has been banned. The ultimate diagnostic tool is the PCR which will readily separate SVD from FMD. On diagnosis in the UK the herd will be slaughtered. The premises will be disinfected with 1% w/v sodium hydroxide and then dried with flame guns. At the present time there is no evidence of the disease in Europe except in Italy.

Teschen Disease

This virus disease, which is thought to be the same as Talfan disease, causes neurological signs. It has never been recorded in the UK and was mainly a disease of Eastern Europe where it was first recorded. It has largely been controlled by vaccination and herd management.

Transmissible Gastroenteritis

TGE is a highly infectious disease of pigs caused by a coronavirus. It is found in England but not in Ireland or Scotland. It is found in the USA and the Far East. It is not found in Australia, New Zealand or Southern Africa. It is monitored by the OIE.

Trichinellosis

This disease is caused by the parasite *Trichinella spiralis*. The larvae live in the muscle of domestic pigs, wild boar and other wild pig species. It is asymptomatic in pigs but causes a very painful condition in man if undercooked infected pork is consumed. As it is a zoonosis it is monitored by the OIE. It is not found in the UK but it is found in mainland Europe, Asia, Africa, North and South America. It is absent from Australia and New Zealand. The main method of transmission is from rats to pigs and then back to rats. It can go direct from pig to pig by cannibalism. Another species, *Trichinella britovi*, is found in foxes. ELISA and random amplification of polymorphic DNA–PCR (RAPD PCR) can be used to diagnose the condition in meat juice. The larvae can be eliminated from the pig by oral dosing with albendazole at 10 mg/kg.

Tularaemia

The bacterium that causes this condition, which is found in man, pigs and many other animals, is called *Francisella tularensis*. It can be spread by aerosol, direct contact, ingestion or arthropods. It occurs in North America, mainland Europe and Asia. It is not found in the UK. In pigs and man it causes acute septicaemia. Diagnosis is by culture and FAT. The main post-mortem sign in pigs is white necrotic foci throughout the liver. The antibiotic of choice for treatment in pigs and man is tetracyclines. At the time of writing there is no vaccine. However, strenuous efforts are being made to make one.

Vesicular Stomatitis

This rare and relatively innocuous viral disease affects cattle, pigs, horses and deer, and extremely rarely man. It was mainly seen on the eastern seaboard of the USA. It is vector spread. Its main importance is that it is clinically similar to FMD.

15 Poisons and Causes of Sudden Death

Mycotoxicosis

Pig feed, particularly cereals, and bedding, e.g. straw, are frequently contaminated with small fungi which produce toxins both while the crop is growing and after it has been harvested and is being stored. The main genera of fungi involved are *Aspergillus* spp., *Claviceps* spp., *Fusarium* spp. and *Penicillin* spp.

These fungi produce a range of toxins under the right conditions for multiplication. Two of these, aflatoxin and ochratoxin, suppress the immune system and also appetite. Growth is retarded. There may be teratogenesis. Fumonisin, another mycotoxin, causes immune suppression but what is more obvious to the clinician is that fumonisin causes pulmonary oedema and resulting respiratory signs. The toxins called trichothecenes, including T-2 and deoxynivalenol (DON), which used to be called vomitoxin, cause gastroenteric signs including weakening of the rectal wall, which may result in rectal prolapse. Zearalenone is an oestrogen-mimicking mycotoxin. It will cause infertility and abortions in sows. Their offspring may well have enlarged vulvas. The famous ergot alkaloids are mycotoxins. They will cause gangrene of the ears, tail and teats.

To control the danger of mycotoxicosis farmers should make sure that mouldy feed is safely discarded and not fed to pigs. It is often fed for economic reasons by unknowing pig keepers or by accident when feed bins have been left and not cleaned properly. Wet straw which has been allowed to dry in bales should not be used as litter for any age of pig.

Plant Poisoning

Introduction

Unlike in grazing farm animals, plant poisoning is rare in pigs. The author has seen very few cases and there are few in the literature.

Arum maculatum

This is known as cuckoo-pint or lords and ladies. It is common throughout England but is rare in Scotland. It has long, dark green leaves with radial stalks. It flowers in May with yellowish-green leaf-like spathes which are 15 cm long. The berries are bright red. It is the white tuberous roots which cause the problem for pigs. They are an intense irritant and cause acute gastritis and vomiting. Later the pig will have intense diarrhoea. Death then follows. There is no specific treatment but demulcents are advised. Euthanasia is probably the most welfare-friendly option.

Beta vulgaris

These are the root family that includes sugar-beet, fodder beet, mangles, turnips, etc. They are not toxic to pigs. Unlike ruminants, pigs do not seem to be affected by excess oxalates. However, problems arise in pigs if these roots are cooked and then allowed to cool in the cooking water. Nitrates and nitrites are released which are toxic. Hb is converted into methaemoglobin, a chocolate-coloured compound which does not exchange oxygen. Pigs go blue, convulse and rapidly die of asphyxia. The known antidote is intravenous methylene blue. In the author's experience this is not successful and euthanasia is advised to prevent further suffering.

Buxus sempervirens

This is box, a common evergreen shrub used as a hedge plant in gardens throughout the UK. It is normally a low hedge but it can be 5 m high. The leaves are elliptical with a notch at the apex. It flowers in April with white flowers. All parts of the plant are toxic. The alkaloid buxine is thought to be the active principle. Pigs are very susceptible to poisoning by box leaves. They vomit and show acute abdominal pain. This is followed by bloody diarrhoea and acute respiratory signs. Death rapidly follows. Treatment is hopeless and prompt euthanasia is indicated.

Conium maculatum

This is hemlock. When consumed in small quantities by sows they give birth to piglets with cleft palates. Normally pigs will not consume sufficient amounts of the plant to cause toxicity.

Daphne mezereum

This is the dwarf bay tree which is sometimes called the spurge olive. It is found in the south of England. It is an erect shrub found in gardens. The flowers are pink and arrive in clusters early in the spring before the leaves. The latter are lanceolate and about 5 cm long. The problem is the red berries, which resemble redcurrants. They are extremely irritant. Only a couple of berries will cause death in a weaner pig. The initial signs are vomiting caused by an acute gastritis. This is followed by collapse and death. The actual toxic substance is not known. There is no specific treatment but demulcents like raw egg and milk are suggested.

Hyoscyamus niger

The universal name for this plant is henbane. It is both an annual and a biennial. It is covered with hairs and has an unpleasant smell. It stands 50 cm high with coarsely lobed, large radial leaves with short stalks. The yellowish-white flowers have a central purple eye. It is the thick, large root which poisons pigs. The active toxins are hyoscyamine, hyoscine and atropine. The plant is found in old monastery gardens where it was grown as a medicine. Pigs will have dilated pupils and dry mouths before going into convulsions. They should be given morphine at 1 mg/10 kg im not only to control the convulsions but also to act as an emetic. There is a chance of recovery if they can be kept warm.

Iris foetidissima

This is the stinking iris which is often called the roast-beef plant. It is found in woodlands throughout the UK. It is an erect perennial plant, 30 cm high, with dark green leaves. It has violet-blue flowers which become bright scarlet seeds. It is the root that causes problems of toxicity in pigs. The pigs will become prostrate and then have violent dysentery. They should be given demulcents as there is normally a chance of recovery.

Lycopersicon esculentum

This is the common tomato and the fruit are not toxic to pigs. However the shoots and stem are toxic. Pigs will be poisoned when rooting in garden rubbish dumps looking for the sweet tomatoes when the whole plants have been discarded. The toxin is solanine. The pigs will be depressed and if they have eaten enough will become laterally recumbent and die. The traditional remedy is strong sweet tea. Ideally this should be given with a teapot slowly into the side of the pig's mouth to avoid inhalation pneumonia. In theory green potatoes should be toxic to pigs as they contain the same toxin. However feeding of greenish potatoes is a very common practice and the author has never seen any evidence of toxicity.

Nicotiana tabacum

The tobacco plant is very toxic to pigs. The active toxin nicotine will cause rapid death if it is digested in relatively small quantities.

Oenanthe crocata

This is water dropwort, also called water hemlock. It is found in marshes throughout the UK. It is a strong perennial plant with a branched hollow stem which has grooves on the outside. It stands 1.5 m high. It has very divided compound leaves. The white flowers, which are umbels, are seen in midsummer. The problem for pigs is the rootstock. These are thick pale yellow tubers, often called 'dead men's fingers'. They are often brought to the surface by dredging or pigs may root them up. The active toxin is oenathetoxin. The roots are still toxic when dried. They are a very potent toxin. Pigs only require a little to go into convulsions, with dilated pupils. Death soon follows. If pigs vomit, there is a chance of recovery. They should be anaesthetized with intravenous barbiturate. This is not easy to administer to a convulsing pig. The author has injected a ketamine anaesthetic cocktail (see Chapter 6) and then topped this up with intravenous barbiturate when the pig is less violent.

Quercus robur

This is the common oak. Pigs are often fed on acorns. However large amounts can cause gastritis. If they are fed acorns with some other feed pigs will show no ill effects. The resulting pork is meant to have more flavour.

Rheum rhaponticum

This is the common garden plant, rhubarb. In theory the leaves, which contain large amounts of oxalates, should be toxic to pigs. However, although the author has seen evidence of pigs eating rhubarb, he has never seen any signs of toxicity. Should practitioners experience this poisoning the antidote is calcium borogluconate. This should only be given iv. The author has seen the results of a subcutaneous injection of a 20% w/v solution of calcium borogluconate mistakenly given by a cowman to a sow with farrowing fever. The majority of the flank of the sow sloughed and the animal had to be destroyed for welfare reasons.

Chemical Poisons

Ammonia

If there is a high level of ammonia in a pig house it is unpleasant for the pig-man and it is equally unpleasant for the pigs, which are nearer the floor. Consistent levels of over 150 ppm will cause reductions in growth rates by a quarter.

Arsenic poisoning

This should be a condition of the past, as arsanilic acid is no longer used in the treatment of swine dysentery. Progressive paralysis and blindness follow tremor. Death follows rapidly.

Pigs will recover if kept warm and given fluids by mouth *ad libitum* (ad lib). As stated earlier, all possible intravenous therapy in pigs is extremely difficult. Sodium thiosulfate can be given by mouth. A suitable dosage would be 10 g for an adult sow; if the pigs have not improved considerably in 3 days, euthanasia should be advised.

Carbadox

If this is included in the diet at three times the therapeutic level there will be reduced food intake and poor growth rates.

Carbon monoxide

Levels of over 50 ppm will cause stillbirths and abortions. Such levels are normally due to faulty gas heaters or motor vehicles running in poorly ventilated buildings.

Cyanide poisoning

In grazing animals cyanide poisoning occurs most frequently from eating plants which contain cyanide. This is not the case in the pig, where the most common poisoning is either from pesticides/rodenticides or from waste chemicals from industrial processes such as metal cleaning. Clinical signs which follow a brief period of excitement are dyspnoea, excess salivation and lacrimation, and vomiting. Muscle fasciculation is seen which becomes generalized spasms, staggering, collapse, coma and death. The mucous membranes are bright red, becoming cyanotic just before death. If pigs survive for over 2 h after the onset of signs, they are likely to recover. Heparinized blood can be analysed to establish a diagnosis before death or liver, preferably frozen on post-mortem, can be stored for analysis later. The consistent post-mortem findings are haemorrhages on liver, lung, heart and trachea. As stated earlier all possible intravenous therapy in pigs is extremely difficult. Sodium thiosulfate can be given by

mouth. A suitable dosage would be 10 g for an adult sow.

Furazolidone

This medicine has been banned in the UK and the EU. It is a fairly toxic medicine. Three times the therapeutic level will cause ataxia and vomiting. Death does not normally occur as the pigs become anorexic.

Iron toxicity

This can occur from the overdosing of injectable iron in piglets. The piglets will be very depressed and will huddle together. Careful examination will normally reveal physical damage to the muscles at the site of injection where a large dose has been injected. There is no specific antidote. Dexamethazone is suggested at 2 mg per piglet injected im. Death usually occurs within 6 h of the iron injection.

Metaldehyde

This is the active ingredient in molluscicides used in the control of snails and slugs. If is often spilt by mistake on farms. It is normally dyed turquoise. It is palatable to pigs.

There is initially excessive salivation. This rapidly leads to inco-ordination and convulsions. Death is then rapid. There is no specific antidote but anaesthetizing the pig ip with barbiturates might be helpful. The hope is that when the pig recovers from the anaesthetic it will have stopped fitting and can make a recovery. The author has had no success with this treatment.

Monensin

Poisoning can occur if pigs eat poultry food. They may be found dead or showing severe neurological signs. The heart will show pale areas on post-mortem. There is no treatment and therefore pigs should be shot if showing severe signs.

Nitrite/nitrate poisoning

This condition has been recorded in pigs which have been fed on whey and are kept in very poorly ventilated conditions. The pigs will initially show subacute respiratory signs making the clinician consider infectious respiratory disease. The distinctive sign is the lack of pyrexia. They do not cough, but just have laboured breathing. They then collapse and become comatose. Normally they will recover if whey is removed from their diet and they are kept warm. Prevention can be carried out by reducing the quantity of whey in the diet and improving the airflow above the pig pens.

Olaquindox

This is a safe medicine but ten times the prescribed level will cause reduction in growth rates.

Organophosphorus poisoning

Organophosphorus poisoning historically was seen as congenital tremor in newborn piglets. This should not be confused with the congenital tremor seen when sows are affected with CSF in late pregnancy. In fact, congenital tremor may be seen after any acute febrile disease e.g. erysipelas suffered by sows in late pregnancy. It is an alarming condition, with the whole litter of piglets violently shaking. It may also be manifest as only a small percentage of the piglets shaking. Often the piglets will survive if they do not shake so much that they cannot hold the teat. Piglets that are shaking badly should be destroyed.

Paraquat

This is an extremely potent poison. Pigs require very little to show toxic signs. There is initial excitement followed by inco-ordination and convulsions. Acute diarrhoea and respiratory distress are very marked. If only small quantities are involved pigs should be injected with a mixture of vitamin E and selenium.

Phenol

Toxicity can occur after the use of these disinfectants if the pigs are introduced when the pens are still wet. Quite severe skin lesions will be apparent. Pigs should be hosed down immediately and any severe burns should be treated with soothing oily creams.

Salt poisoning

This really is water deprivation and is one of the most common causes of neurological signs in growing pigs. It occurs if the water supply is turned off or frozen up. A growing pig weighing 15 kg requires 2 l of water per day. Pigs do not like to wait for water and it is very important that there is a ready supply available to them. This is important when the piglets are still suckling the sow. A 100 kg finishing pig requires 12 l daily. Pigs do not like to queue so adequate nipple drinkers of clean fresh water should be available. Neurological signs are more prominent in growing pigs. When the supply of water is reinstated the water should be controlled. In severely affected pigs, dexamethasone injections will help with recovery.

Selenium poisoning

This is extremely rare. The author has seen the condition in pigs which were given a large amount of an equine supplement. The fattening pigs remained mentally alert but were reluctant to rise. In fact they appeared unable to rise for 12 h. There was no specific antidote available. They recovered with careful nursing.

Warfarin

Pigs will consume rat bait containing warfarin. The signs of toxicity are coughing up blood, bloody diarrhoea and haemorrhages visible in the skin. Aggressive treatment with intramuscular injections of vitamin K will normally be successful.

Reactions to Medicines

Penicillin

If procaine penicillin is inadvertently injected iv, pigs will show immediate trembling. They will recover in a few hours without treatment.

Tiamulin

Rarely tiamulin, if fed at standard therapeutic levels for the treatment of swine dysentery, will cause adverse reactions. These may be just a slight reddening or in extremely rare cases death will occur. In these cases haemorrhages will be seen in the myocardium.

Causes of Sudden Death

Iatrogenic causes of sudden death

Sudden death is a misnomer. In reality it is found dead since last seen. The owner will very rarely see an animal die. It is even rarer for the clinician to see death. Sadly when such deaths occur it is usually at the time of veterinary treatment. Possible iatrogenic causes of sudden death are:

- Anaphylaxis from administration of medicines.
- General anaesthesia.
- Restraint leading to cardiac arrest.
- Lumbar/sacral epidural.
- Massive haemorrhage (this could occur at parturition where there is no human involvement).

- Intra-arterial injection.
- Intravenous injection.
- Sedation.

Reasons for animals to be found dead

African swine fever

It is unlikely that every pig will be found dead. The sick animals will have had an extremely high rectal temperature which drops before the clinical signs of marked cyanosis of the skin and inco-ordination develop. There will be severe haemorrhages throughout the body, particularly in the lymph nodes. Tissue or body fluids can be used to demonstrate antibody. Frozen sections of tissue may be used to demonstrate virus which may also be isolated from cultures of buffy coat leucocytes. The ultimate diagnostic tool is animal transmission.

Anthrax

Pigs found dead are not the normal manifestation of anthrax except in young pigs. Older animals will show throat swelling. Samples of this throat swelling should be collected to prepare slides for staining with methylene blue. The spleen may be enlarged but this is not an invariable finding.

Aujeszky's disease

Sudden death will occur only in young pigs. Older pigs will show neurological signs. Adults may show few signs. There will be few gross post-mortem findings. Virus may be isolated from frozen tonsil section. PCR may be used on fixed tonsil, brain or nasal swabs.

Bowel oedema

This is a disease of newly weaned pigs. Some of the litter may be found dead. The remainder will have the characteristic oedema of eyelids, larynx, etc. The post-mortem will reveal excess peritoneal, pleural and pericardial fluid. The isolation of specific *Escherichia coli* serotypes from the small intestine will aid diagnosis.

Chemical poisons

These will show variable post-mortem pictures. They are itemized above.

Classical swine fever

Only in the hyperacute disease will some young pigs be found dead. Other pigs will show high fever and conjunctivitis. Post-mortem may not show any gross lesions in the hyperacute cases but less acute cases will show a haemorrhagic skin and internally the lymph nodes will be very inflamed. There are splenic infarcts. Virus can be demonstrated by FAT on frozen sections of the tonsil. Virus may also be demonstrated from RT-PCR from the lymph nodes. Serology using ELISAs will be helpful, with animal transmission as the final definitive test.

Clostridiosis

This will cause sudden death in baby pigs with the characteristic 'port wine-coloured diarrhoea'. There will also be sudden death in adults and large fat pigs. There is rapid decomposition of the carcass. There is tracheal froth and pulmonary oedema. There is an 'Aero chocolate' liver. *Clostridium novyi* may be identified in the liver with FAT or PCR.

Coliform mastitis

This will cause sudden death only in newly farrowed sows. The glands will be swollen and hard without any secretion. The organism may be cultured from an infected gland.

Cystitis/pyelonephritis

Cystitis will not cause sudden death and in fact pyelonephritis will very rarely cause acute symptoms. Sudden death occurs only when both kidneys are affected from an ascending infection from cystitis with a toxic *E. coli* strain. Post-mortem will reveal the infected kidneys.

Drowning

Pigs can swim but they will get cold and exhausted (Fig. 15.1). The lungs will be waterlogged on post-mortem and will sink if placed in water.

Erysipelas/endocarditis

Endocarditis will cause sudden death. If there is left-sided heart failure there will be fluid pooling in the tissues and peritoneum. If there is right-side heart failure there will be fluid in the lungs and thorax. Cyanosis will be a feature in right-side heart failure.

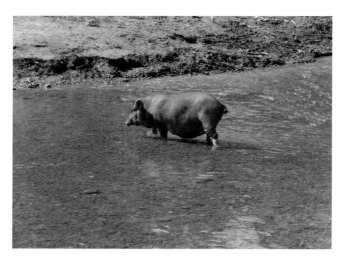

Fig. 15.1. Pigs can swim.

Electrocution

It is vital to turn off the electricity supply before examining the pigs. The diagnosis will be made on circumstantial evidence. The heart muscle will show streaks of haemorrhage. At least one post-mortem should be performed in case there is an insurance claim.

Encephalomyocarditis

This is caused by a cardiovirus. The virus is much more common in tropical areas in cattle. It will cause sudden death in young pigs. The whole carcass will be congested with large amounts of fluid in the body cavities. The heart will be soft and pale with some totally white areas. The virus may be demonstrated by RT-PCR from the myocardial cells.

Gassing from slurry

The diagnosis will be made from circumstantial evidence. The whole carcass will be congested. There will be cyanosis. The lungs will be congested and the pleural cavity full of fluid.

Gastric/splenic torsion

This condition is seen in adults and occasionally in large fat pigs. The pig will appear bloated. The torsion can readily be diagnosed on post-mortem.

Heat stroke

This is normally a condition of white pigs outside with no shade or water to cool in. The carcass will be very red and congested.

Haemophilus infection

This infection will cause sudden death in growing and fattening pigs. Normally the infection affects the respiratory and circulatory systems and so there is congestion throughout the carcass. The abdomen may also be affected. The diagnosis can be confirmed by culture. There may well be other pathogens involved.

Hertztod

This condition is another variant of the porcine stress syndrome (PSS). Diagnosis is difficult. Genetic susceptibility will give an idea of a diagnosis.

Intestinal haemorrhage syndrome

This is the same as whey bloat described below.

Intestinal volvulus/intussusception/intestinal foreign body/hernial entrapment

These are causes of sudden death only if the pigs have not been observed carefully over the previous 12 h. The diagnosis is obvious on post-mortem.

Leptospirosis

This is not a likely cause of sudden death. In theory, a pig suffering from the septicaemic form with acute liver failure might be found dead. The carcass will be jaundiced. Histological sections of the liver and kidney will show the organisms when stained with a silver stain.

Lightening strike

This is an extremely rare cause of sudden death in pigs. It is over-diagnosed as it is one of the few conditions covered by farmers' insurance. There must have been a thunderstorm. This can be verified on the internet. The pigs need to be outside and touching a fence or pig ark. Haemorrhage streaks are meant to be seen in the subcutaneous tissues on the forelegs. These rarely can be found. Practitioners may make the diagnosis on circumstantial evidence.

Malignant hyperthermia

This condition certainly causes sudden death in growing and adult pigs. It is all part of the PSS described below.

Mulberry heart disease

Classically this cause of sudden death occurs in large fattening pigs but it can occur in any age of pig. There are pericardial and endocardial streaky haemorrhages. The liver is large and mottled. The vitamin E levels in the liver can be used to confirm the diagnosis.

Pasteurellosis

This is a common condition but rarely causes sudden death. Sudden death is seen only in growing pigs with a peracute pneumonia with cardiac involvement. There will be obvious post-mortem signs and the organism may be cultured to confirm the diagnosis.

Poisonous plants

This is a rare cause of sudden death as not only is plant poisoning rare in pigs, but also few plants cause sudden death. The plants are described above.

Porcine dermatitis and nephropathy syndrome

PDNS will cause sudden death in large fat pigs and occasionally in adults. The skin on the rear end of the pig will have large purple patches. There is pneumonia and a generalized lymphadenopathy. The kidneys are enlarged. Histology of the kidney may help to confirm the disease, which resembles CSF.

Porcine stress syndrome

PSS, which causes sudden death, is part of an inherited disease complex which includes malignant hyperthermia and pale soft exudative muscle. Rigor mortis develops rapidly. The pale areas of muscle are easily seen on post-mortem both in skeletal and cardiac muscle. There is a PCR test to show the presence of genetic susceptibility.

Post-weaning multisytemic wasting syndrome

PMWS is not a cause of sudden death, although chronically affected animals may well be found dead. The carcass will be extremely emaciated. The lungs do not collapse and the liver is atrophic.

Proliferative haemorrhagic enteropathy

PHE may cause sudden death in growing pigs. The carcass will be pale. The small intestine, mainly the lower third, will be distended and filled with a mixture of food and blood. The causal organism can be identified in smears to confirm the diagnosis.

Ruptured aneurysm

This can be a mysterious cause of sudden death in any age of pig if the ruptured aneurysm is in the brain. In adult pigs the aneurysm which ruptures may be in the abdomen, so the carcass will be pale and the abdomen full of blood.

Ruptured uterine artery

This causes sudden death in sows at parturition. The carcass will be pale and the abdomen full of blood.

Salmonellosis

This is not a normal cause of sudden death except the septicaemic form in young pigs. There is discoloration of the skin and ears. The lymph nodes are large and haemorrhagic. The spleen is enlarged. The organism can be cultured to confirm the diagnosis.

Septic metritis

This can cause sudden death immediately after parturition, particularly if there has been a large amount of intervention. Death is caused by a toxin-producing *E. coli*. There will be a smelly vulval discharge and the vulva will be blue. The septic uterus will be seen on post-mortem.

Snake bite

The author has seen this only in an outdoor sow in Western Australia. The double fang marks were clearly visible on the white snout. The species of snake was unknown.

Streptococcal infections

The meningitis caused by these organisms in newly weaned pigs is unlikely to cause sudden death. On the other hand, sudden death in large fattening pigs is the norm. The organism can usually be cultured from the heart blood so that removal of the brain is unnecessary.

Teschen/Talfan disease

This neurological viral condition has been recorded as being peracute and causing sudden death in central Europe. It is not found in the UK. Diagnosis would be with histology of the brain.

Thiamin deficiency

This causes myocardial degeneration. It is seen in pigs fed on an all-bread diet or fed large quantities of bracken.

Trauma

For trauma to be severe enough in a pig to cause sudden death, a motor vehicle would need to be involved. The author has seen a bush pig killed by a train in Kenya.

Uterine prolapse

If the middle uterine artery has been ruptured, this condition will cause sudden death.

Uterine rupture

This is unlikely to cause sudden death. Sows will be found dead after a difficult farrowing and a uterine rupture.

Whey bloat

This causes sudden death in large fattening pigs. They will be pale and bloated. The small intestine will be swollen and contain blood-stained fluid.

16 Zoonotic Diseases

Introduction

Zoonotic diseases have always been important. However, they are even more important now as the number of emerging diseases with zoonotic implications is increasing rapidly. Veterinarians have a large role to play in controlling these diseases and in advising their medical colleagues on the real risks that animal diseases pose to man. Zoonotic diseases can be viral, bacterial, fungal, protozoal and parasitic in origin. Veterinarians are uniquely qualified to advise on prevention and reduce the chances of transmission to humans by proper education and management techniques. Veterinarians have a duty of care to the general populace, to the owners of the animals concerned, to their own staff and of course to themselves. Washable protective clothing should be worn if possible.

There are some very simple measures which can be taken to protect yourself, your family and your staff from zoonotic diseases. You can also advise your clients how to protect themselves and their families as well as visitors to their farms:

- Never eat undercooked pig meat.
- Never cuddle newly born piglets or give mouth-to-mouth resuscitation.
- Always wash your hands thoroughly after handling pigs.
- Always wash your hands before handling food.
- Remove dirty clothes before entering the kitchen.
- Pay particular attention to the hygiene of children.
- Keep the farm clean.
- Keep pigs, their feed and water clean.
- Handle dung, manure, slurry and sewage safely.
- Protect water supplies and watercourses.
- Reduce transport stress of animals.
- Keep transport vehicles clean.

Viral Zoonotic Diseases Found in Pigs Categorized by Their Human Medical Name

Crimean–Congo haemorrhagic fever

This is a systemic disease affecting the blood vessels caused by a nairovirus and spread by ticks. It is found in pigs as well as in cattle, sheep and goats in Central Asia, Bulgaria and the Congo.

Encephalomyocarditis

This is a neurological and cardiac disease caused by a cardiovirus and called three-day fever. It is found in pigs but more commonly in cattle. It is extremely rarely transmitted from animals to man. However, as pigs are kept more intensively and in closer proximity to man they are a more likely source.

Foot and mouth disease

FMD is a benign disease in man caused by an aphthovirus. It is the most contagious disease found in cattle, sheep, goats, South American camelids (SACs) and pigs known to veterinary science. There are rigorous control measures in place for its control. The disease has a rare incidence nowadays. Even in widespread pandemics in the past, cases seen in man were extremely rare. Man potentially can harbour the virus in the upper airway for 3 days after contact.

Influenza

This is a well-known generalized systemic disease caused by a variety of influenza viruses that is sometimes called grippe. It occurs in man worldwide. It is also found worldwide in pigs. Normally pig viruses are not infective to man. However, on occasions there are mutations so that pigs living in close contact to man will infect their keepers. On account of air travel such viruses soon occur in other countries. The human vaccines are regularly updated.

Japanese B encephalitis

This is a severe neurological disease caused by a flavivirus, which is spread in man by mosquitoes. It is found in pigs in India and the Far East. There is cross-infection between pigs and man by mosquitoes but this is rare.

Rabies

This a fatal neurological disease caused by a lyssavirus. It causes acute encephalitis both in man and animals and the pig is no exception. It is usually transmitted to humans by a bite from a carnivore. However, pigs can also transmit the disease by biting not only other pigs but in-contact humans. It is almost invariably fatal in man if post-exposure prophylaxis is not administered before the onset of severe symptoms.

The condition has been known for more than 4000 years. In the 4th century BC, Aristotle warned of the danger of being bitten by a rabid dog. In 1821, Francois Magendie, in France, showed that a dog would develop rabies if inoculated with saliva from a human case (Brightman, 2012). It was not until the 1880s that Louis Pasteur produced a successful vaccine.

The rabies virus is the most common rhabdovirus to infect man. It is readily destroyed by exposure to sunlight and by boiling. It is less easily destroyed by disinfectants. The virus is excreted in the saliva of infected pigs and other animals, including man. Excretion may occur 48 h before there are signs of the disease.

Rabies is found in most parts of the world except in the UK, Scandinavia, Australia and New Zealand. At least 100,000 people die each year from rabies, mostly in India and the Far East, in particular Thailand (Brightman, 2012). Rabies has been eliminated from domestic animals in countries such as the USA, so wild animals such as racoons are reservoirs of infection. In South America, vampire bats transmit rabies to pigs and sometimes to man.

Animals vary in their susceptibility to rabies. Wolves and foxes are very susceptible, whereas dogs are less so and wild boar and pigs even less so.

After a bite the virus enters the body and disappears rapidly from the site of inoculation, spreading to the brain by retrograde axoplasmic flow through the peripheral nerves. Once it has become established in the brain, it spreads back to the peripheral tissues through the nervous system. The incubation in pigs is similar to that in man. It is normally between 1 and 3 months, but a time of over a year has been recorded.

In pigs the most common form of rabies is the 'furious' form with the pig attacking any other animal on sight. This is particularly alarming in wild boar and bush pigs. The 'dumb' form where the rabid pig hides is more common in warthogs and giant forest hogs but less common in domestic pigs.

Diagnosis can be carried out in the live pig with a PCR on saliva, but more commonly the diagnosis is made by the finding of the pathognomic demonstration of Negri bodies in the cells of the hippocampus.

In very rare cases successful treatment has been carried out in man. Euthanasia should be carried out in pigs without damaging the brain, so that diagnosis can be confirmed.

Rotaviral gastroenteritis

There is a gastroenteric disease of children caused by a rotavirus. The virus found in suckling pigs worldwide is a different virus. However, if children receive a massive dose of the pig virus they will show diarrhoea. Normal hygiene procedures are important.

Swine influenza

In 2009, the world witnessed the rapid spread of an influenza A virus of the H1N1 subtype, namely A(H1N1)pdm09, through the human population. Although this virus was not identified in animals before its emergence in human beings, genetic studies strongly suggest that pigs were the putative host species (Smith *et al.*, 2009). Subsequently, the reverse process occurred as A(H1N1)-pdm09 transmitted back from human beings into and within the global pig population (Sims, 2012).

These pig viruses readily spread in pig populations. The virus can be transmitted from infected breeding herds, displaying no or few signs, to other herds that purchase piglets from these farms. Active surveillance is therefore very important to protect both the human and the pig population. The failure to detect the 2009 human pandemic strain in pigs before it crossed the species barrier demonstrated major deficiencies in global influenza surveillance in pigs.

Swine vesicular disease

This is a mild disease in man caused by an enterovirus. It is very rare in man and is extremely rare in pigs worldwide. It is very rarely zoonotic. It is important in pigs as clinically it cannot be differentiated from FMD.

Vesicular stomatitis

This disease is called 'sore mouth' in man. It is caused by a vesiculovirus. It affects pigs in North and South America. It is a mild disease in man and is extremely rarely zoonotic.

Bacterial Zoonotic Diseases Found in Pigs Categorized by Their Human Medical Name

Animal erysipelas (human erysipeloid)

There is considerable confusion concerning this condition as a zoonosis. The zoonosis is caused by the bacterium *Erysipelothrix rhusiopathiae*. This organism is found in the soil all over the world. It commonly causes disease in pigs. It will infect man through wounds from the skin disease in pigs. Veterinary surgeons, abattoir workers and pig keepers are most at risk. The disease is readily treated with penicillin.

The confusion arises as there is a condition in man termed erysipelas by the medical profession. This is commonly called 'fish-sorters' disease'. It is not caused by *E. rhusiopathiae* but by a streptococcus. This organism is found in fish and in marine mammals.

Anthrax

This disease is caused by *Bacillus anthracis* which occurs in all mammals worldwide. It has three manifestations in man. 'Wool-sorters' disease' is the invariably fatal pneumonic form caught from the skins of sheep and goats.

There is an enteric form from eating carcasses contaminated with *B. anthracis*. This enteric form is the normal method of transfer of anthrax from pigs to man. The third form which can be transmitted between pigs and man is the skin form.

Botulism

This disease is caused by the toxin produced by the anaerobic spore-forming bacterium, *Clostridium botulinum*. All warm-blooded animals are affected. Botulism is normally not an actual zoonosis as man is poisoned by eating food in which the bacterium has produced toxin, e.g. in contaminated fish. Cases have been recorded worldwide. However if pig carcasses contaminated by the toxin are consumed they will cause death.

Brucellosis

Brucella suis is found in pigs worldwide but not in the UK or Northern Europe. It is extremely rarely zoonotic.

Campylobacteriosis

This disease is caused by *Campylobacter jejuni*. It is the main cause of acute bacterial enteritis in the UK. The most common animal host to be a danger to man is the chicken. It is also found in pigs worldwide but is extremely rarely zoonotic.

Clostridial food poisoning

Although these many species of bacteria are very important and prevalent in all farm animals, it is not an important zoonosis. The organism is found in soil and dust worldwide and so animals are not the main cause of infection. The clostridial spp. that occur in pigs cause very mild enteritis in man which rarely lasts more than 24 h. It is self-limiting. The important pathogen in man is *Clostridium*

difficile, which is not pathogenic in pigs, nor is it found in them.

Colibacillosis

This is a very important life-threatening zoonotic disease found worldwide. The most important highly pathogenic *Escherichia coli* in the UK is the verocytotoxigenic strain *E. coli* O157. In other countries there are other verocytotoxigenic strains e.g. O26. Verocytotoxigenic strain *E. coli* (VTEC) O157 is carried asymptomatically by animals and owners of animals should be aware of the potential for zoonotic transmission of VTEC O157 even from healthy animals. It is very rarely found in pigs. It is much more common in herbivores. The organism colonizes the rectal-anal junction of pigs with certain individuals being supershedders. General hygiene precautions are important.

Enterocolitic yersiniosis

This serious disease is caused by *Yersinia enterocolitica*. It occurs in pigs worldwide. However, pigs are very rarely important as a disease source for man. Rodents are the main hazard and they need to be controlled to reduce the disease in man and pigs.

Leptospirosis

There is considerable confusion with this worldwide zoonotic disease. *Leptospira icterohaemorrhagiae* causes a very serious, often fatal disease in man, called 'Weil's disease'. This disease is passed to man from rodents which are normally symptomless carriers. Pigs can get the disease from rodents or other pigs and infect man. There are other *Leptospira* serovars which can also affect pigs and are a potential zoonotic threat. Actually, pigs are extremely rarely implicated in infections in humans. Infected water is a much larger hazard. Cattle will become infected with *Leptospira harjo*. This serovar can infect pigs but it is rare. *L. harjo* is not a cause of serious disease in man.

Listeriosis

This worldwide disease is caused by *Listeria monocytogenes*. It is a very serious infection in very young babies and will cause abortion in women. It is commonly found in pigs. In some countries up to 10% of pig herds may be affected. It is normally isolated from the tonsil but most infections are asymptomatic. In rare cases baby piglets die. Pigs are extremely rarely the cause of a zoonotic infection.

Meliodosis

This disease is caused by *Burkholderia pseudomallei* and is also called rodent glanders. It is mainly confined to pigs in the tropics, particularly South-east Asia. Normally it is asymptomatic in pigs, although cases showing symptoms have been reported. Pigs will be pyrexic with marked swelling of the limbs. The carcass is full of abscesses. Culture is diagnostic. It is an extremely severe disease in man which is often fatal. Excellent hygiene precautions should be adopted.

Pasteurellosis

Pasteurella multocida causes widespread pneumonia problems worldwide in pigs. *Mannheimia haemolytica* is rare in pigs and normally is associated with close contact with infected sheep. Deaths in growing pigs have been reported. Both organisms have been recorded as zoonoses but they are extremely rarely related to pigs.

Salmonellosis

Salmonella typhimurium is a common pathogen in pigs in the UK, Europe and worldwide. It will cause enteritis in man but infection from pigs is rarely implicated. *Salmonella enteritidis* is found mainly in poultry worldwide and will cause enteritis in man. *S. enteritidis* is rarely found in pigs. *Salmonella dublin* is found mainly in cattle and rarely causes enteritis in man. It is rarely found in pigs. *Salmonella choleraesuis* is mainly a pig pathogen and very rarely infects man. There are other causes of salmonellosis which are ever present on farms, e.g. *Salmonella enterica* sbsp. *diarizonae* and *Salmonella montevideo*. These will infect man and pigs but the infection rarely comes from pigs.

Most human salmonella infections are acquired as a result of eating contaminated food. Infection on farms is more commonly acquired by mouth from hands contaminated by infected animals, their bedding and surroundings. The following simple precautions will go a long way to prevent people associated with livestock from becoming infected with salmonellosis.

- Do observe high standards of personal hygiene; wear rubber boots and protective over-garments when working with animals.
- Do change and launder overalls frequently and disinfect boots to avoid spreading the infection to other animals and people.
- Do wash your hands using hot water and soap immediately after working with infected animals.
- Do wash hands before eating, drinking or smoking.
- Do ensure that anyone with diarrhoea, vomiting or flu-like illness consults a doctor, and informs the doctor if salmonellas have been isolated from livestock.
- Do not take or wear dirty clothing and boots into the home.
- Do not allow vulnerable people, including children, the elderly and pregnant women, to come into contact with infected animals.
- Do not bring infected animals into any room where food is prepared or eaten.
- Do not allow pets to come in contact with infected animals.

Cleaning and disinfection are vital for the control of salmonellosis as with most other bacterial and indeed viral diseases. However with salmonellosis it is important to have a specific herd health plan for this disease.

To encourage compliance the use of a 'before-and-after' swabbing system is useful. Specifically designed swabs should be used to identify the presence of both salmonella and enterobacteria. These swabs taken from the floor and walls can be cultured in 24 h. They will show the presence of both groups of bacteria.

There are no shortcuts when carrying out an effective cleaning and disinfection routine. The main rule is that there should be a three-phase process. This must include thorough cleaning, then disinfection followed by thorough drying. Cleaning should be dry mechanically initially followed by hand finishing. This should be followed by wet cleaning which should include not only suitable detergents but also clean water. The surfaces must then be dried or the disinfectant to then be used will be diluted below its approved level. After the required time the disinfectant should be washed off with clean water and then it is vital that the whole pen is totally dried. The longer the pens can be left vacant after drying the better.

Fungal Zoonotic Diseases Found in Pigs Categorized by Their Human Medical Name

Dermatophytosis

Compared with cattle, ringworm in pigs is extremely rare. They will contract *Trichophyton verrucosum* from cattle. In theory they could then be contagious to man.

Protozoal Zoonotic Diseases Found in Pigs Categorized by Their Human Medical Name

Sarcocystosis

The disease in pigs is caused by *Sarcocystis suihominis*. Man is usually a symptomless carrier. The disease occurs worldwide. It is an extremely rare zoonosis.

Parasitic Zoonotic Diseases Found in Pigs Categorized by Their Human Medical Name

Acanthocephaliasis

This disease is caused by the nematode *Macracanthorhynchus hirudinaceus*, which occurs in the small intestine of man and pigs in Eastern Europe and Asia. It is avoided by normal hygiene precautions.

Ascariasis

There are two species of ascarid nematode which are very similar, *Ascaris lumbricoides* in man and *Ascaris suum* in pigs. They can rarely infect the heterologous host. Therefore *A. suum* is rarely thought of as a zoonosis. They are both found worldwide.

Clonorchiasis

This disease is caused by a fluke, *Clonorchis sinensis*. It affects man and pigs. It has two intermediate hosts, a snail and a fish. It occurs in the Far East.

Echinostomiasis

This disease is caused by several species of fluke of the genus *Echinostoma* found in the Far East. It has two intermediate hosts, a snail and then another snail, a tadpole or a fish. Man, pigs and poultry, particularly ducks and geese, are infected by eating the second intermediate host. Pigs are very rarely implicated.

Gastrodiscoidiasis

The disease-causing fluke, *Gastrodiscoides hominis*, occurs in man and pigs and has a single intermediate host, an aquatic snail. It occurs in Asia.

Taeniasis and cysticercosis

The cestode *Taenia solium* has man as the definitive host. The secondary host is the pig, which has the larval stages of *Cysticercus cellulosae*. Normally man is infected with *T. solium* from eating pig meat. Self re-infection can occur. The parasite is now rare but is recorded worldwide.

Trichinosis

This disease is caused by a small filiform nematode, *Trichinella spiralis*. Man is the end host and is infected by eating undercooked pig meat. The pig can be both the intermediate and main host. The disease occurs rarely in North and South America and extremely rarely elsewhere. It is not found in the UK.

The bush pig is the intermediate host in Eastern and Southern Africa.

Tungiasis

This condition which occurs in pigs and man is caused by a small flea, *Tunga penetrans*. It occurs in tropical areas of Africa, the Caribbean, Central and South America.

Zoonotic scabies

This disease, scabies, is caused by a mite, *Sarcoptes scabiei*. A very similar mite is found in pigs which can infect humans. Man is extremely rarely infected by pigs and human infections usually are caught from other humans. It is found worldwide.

Appendix: Veterinary Medicines

Pig Medicines

Introduction

In the UK there are medicines which are specifically licensed for use in pigs. Under a code of conduct called the cascade principle these licensed medicines must be used first to treat any condition. If they are not effective or if there is no specifically licensed product available, then a clinician may prescribe a medicine licensed for another species. Some of these medicines are recorded at the end of this chapter. If there is no product licensed for animals but there is a product licensed for human use this can then be used. At the time of writing the author has never needed to prescribe a product licensed for human medicine. The cascade principle is a long-standing legal flexibility providing a rational balance between the legislative requirement for veterinary surgeons to prescribe and use authorized veterinary medicines where they are available, and the need for professional freedom to prescribe other products where they are not. It is intended to increase the range of medicines available for veterinary use. The medicines available in the UK are listed below under the headings: (i) anti-inflammatory preparations (both injectable and oral); (ii) antimicrobial preparations (both injectable and oral); (iii) cardiovascular and respiratory preparations (both injectable and oral); (iv) dietary supplements and fluid metabolites (both injectable and oral); (v) antiparasitic preparations (both injectable and oral); and (vi) other medicines. Dosages and meat withhold times are all recorded. Medicines for inclusion into food are not included. Practitioners are urged to consult the latest handbook of feed additives.

Practitioners from the EU will be familiar with these medicines listed below as they are in the main licensed throughout the EU. The generic name of the drug is given to ease understanding for practitioners both in Europe and the rest of the world.

Medicine care on-farm

In addition to the appropriate selection of medicines, it is vital that veterinary surgeons on-farm also provide advice on the security, storage, hygiene, use and disposal of pharmaceutical products (Carr and Smith, 2013). It is important that standard operating procedures are in place to fulfil these criteria. On large commercial pig farms reviewing the use of medicines is an essential part of any herd health maintenance programme. It is also important that practitioners guide keepers of backyard pigs on the safe use of veterinary medicines. This is particularly important as there is likely to be a large amount of owner medication and also the pigs are likely to be kept in a home/family environment. Medicines must be placed in a secure location away from children, animals and thieves. They must be in a lockable storage facility. Vaccines and certain medicines need to be kept refrigerated at a temperature between 2°C and 8°C. The vaccines should not be over-stocked or the correct temperature will not be maintained. Also the door should not be opened too often. This fridge should be kept locked. Medicines should not be stored in a fridge used to store food. The temperature of the fridge should be monitored regularly with the use of a maximum and minimum thermometer.

Health and safety

Certain products may need to be kept more securely, so that if the bottle falls and breaks the medication does not come in contact with human skin. Prostaglandins are a classic example. Needles need to be disposed of in a dedicated sharps container. This can be a labelled Coke can on smallholdings which can be given to the practitioner for safe disposal. Needles should not be left in bottles.

When bottles have been breached the date should be recorded on the side of the bottle. The bottle then must be disposed of after the time specified on the bottle. Staff suffering from accidents involving veterinary medicines should seek medical attention. This action should be recorded in a dedicated bound book labelled 'Accident book'.

Anti-inflammatory preparations

These preparations are very useful in pigs to control pain by relieving inflammation. They are best given at the same time as antimicrobials. There is some debate as to their length of action. The data sheets would indicate that this is only 24 h. However many practitioners consider they will last longer, particularly meloxicam. Table A.1 includes the only licensed products which are available in the UK at the time of writing. The generic ingredients are

given for use by practitioners in other countries. On the whole NSAIDs should be used in preference to corticosteroids, which have more side-effects. Corticosteroids should never be given to pregnant animals. Most injectable NSAIDs have a short meat withhold period except for flunixin meglumine. Dexamethazone has a very variable withhold period. Clinicians should utilize the preparations with short withhold periods if slaughter is imminent. Oral sodium salicylate has a zero withhold period, but oral paracetamol has a withhold of 28 days.

Antimicrobial preparations

Tables A.2 (injectables), A.3 (oral products to be used in the feed or drinking water), A.4 (oral products to be given directly by mouth) and A.5 (topical products) include the only licensed antimicrobial products which are available in the UK at the time of writing. The generic ingredients are given for use of practitioners in other countries. The clinician needs to make sure the antimicrobial is suitable for the infection being treated. Then it is important to discuss with the pig keeper the mode of administration. Unweaned pigs will need to be treated by individual injections for most infections, except for enteric infections which need to be treated by mouth using a specially designed 'pig-pump'. Lactating sows will normally be treated by injection. However follow-up treatment could be oral in the food or water. Groups of sows, gilts, fattening and growing pigs can be treated in the water or in the food. Obviously an anorexic pig should not be treated in the food; however, often such pigs will be drinking so that water medication may be appropriate. Clinicians must be aware that injectable antimicrobial treatment is likely to give the highest blood levels but the difficulty in treatment, particularly in outside pigs, may make this very difficult.

Clinicians must always be aware of withhold periods. These tend to be long with penicillins and oxytetracyclines but much shorter with cephalosporins. Withhold periods should be strictly adhered to on account

Table A.1. Anti-inflammatory preparations, both injectable and oral.

Medicine	Active substance	Dose	Meat withhold (days)
Comforion Vet 100 mg/ml Solution for Injection for Horse, Cattle and Swine	100 mg ketoprofen/ml	1 ml/33 kg im daily	4
Dexadreson	2 mg dexamethasone/ml	1.5 ml/50 kg iv or im once and repeated in 48 h	2
Emdocam 20 mg/ml Injection	20 mg meloxicam/ml	2 ml/100 kg im daily for two injections	5
Finadyne Solution	50 mg flunixin meglumine/ml	2 ml/45 kg im	22
Flunixin Injection	50 mg flunixin meglumine/ml	2 ml/45 kg im	22
Ketodale 100 mg/ml Solution for Injection for Horses, Cattle and Swine	100 mg ketoprofen/ml	3 ml/100 kg im	4
Ketofen 10%	100 mg ketoprofen/ml	3 ml/100 kg im	4
Melovem 5 mg/ml Solution for Injection for Cattle and Pigs	5 mg meloxicam/ml	2 ml/25 kg im daily for two injections	5
Meloxidyl 20 mg/ml Solution for Injection for Cattle, Pigs and Horses	20 mg meloxicam/ml	2 ml/100 kg im daily for two injections	5
Metacam 20 mg/ml Solution for Injection for Cattle, Pigs and Horses	20 mg meloxicam/ml	2 ml/100 kg im daily for two injections	5
Pracetam	200 mg paracetamol/ml solution or 200 mg paracetamol/g powder	1.5 mg/10 kg daily for 5 days (unlicensed in the UK)	28
Rapidexon	2 mg dexamethasone/ml	1.5 ml/50 kg iv or im once and repeated in 48 h	2
Rheumocam 20 mg/ml Injection for Cattle, Pigs and Horses	20 mg meloxicam/ml	2 ml/100 kg im	5
Sodium Salicyl 80% WSP Powder for Oral for Cattle (Calves) and Pigs	800 mg sodium salicylate/g	35 mg sodium salicylate/kg for 3–5 days	0
Solacyl Oral Powder	1000 mg sodium salicylate/g	35 mg/kg orally in drinking water for 3–5 days	0
Tolfine	4 mg tolfenamic acid/ml	1 ml/20 kg im as a single injection	3
Voren Suspension for Injection, 1 mg/ml	1 mg dexamethazone/ml	2 ml/100 kg im in growing pigs and adults; 1 ml/10 kg im in piglets	55

of human health. It is vital that practising veterinary surgeons play their part in the careful use of antimicrobials to avoid the build-up of antimicrobial resistance. This is particularly important with the in-feed use of antimicrobials, which should be replaced by good husbandry practices, including vaccination. Antimicrobials have been banned in the EU for growth-promoting purposes.

Table A.2. Antimicrobials (injectables).

Medicine	Active substance	Dose	Meat withhold (days)
Advocin 2.5% Solution for Injection	25 mg danofloxacin/ml	1 ml/20 kg im daily	3
Alamycin 10	100 mg oxytetracycline/ml	1 ml/11–50 kg im daily	20
Alamycin LA	200 mg oxytetracycline/ml	1 ml/10 kg im as a single injection	18
Alamycin LA 300	300 mg oxytetracycline/ml	1 ml/10–15 kg im as a single injection	14–28 (depending on dosage)
Amfipen LA	100 mg ampicillin/ml	1 ml/4 kg im every 2 days	60
Amoxycare Injection	150 mg amoxicillin/ml	1 ml/21 kg im daily	16
Amoxycare LA Injection	150 mg amoxicillin/ml	1 ml/10 kg im every 2 days	16
Amoxypen Injection	150 mg amoxicillin/ml	1 ml/20 kg im daily	16
Amoxypen LA	150 mg amoxicillin/ml	1 ml/10 kg im daily	16
Baytril 5% Solution for Injection	50 mg enrofloxacin/ml	2.5 ml/100 kg im daily (this dose rate may be doubled for treating salmonellosis and complicated respiratory disease)	10
Baytril 10% Solution for Injection	100 mg enrofloxacin/ml	0.5 ml/10 kg im daily (this dose rate may be doubled for treating salmonellosis and complicated respiratory disease)	10
Baytril Max	100 mg enrofloxacin/ml	0.75 ml/10 kg im as a single dose	
Betamox Injection	150 mg amoxicillin/ml	1 ml/21 kg im daily	16
Betamox LA	150 mg amoxicillin/ml	1 ml/10 kg im every 2 days	16
Cefenil Powder and Solvent Solution for Injection	1 g ceftiofur/20 ml	1 ml/50 kg im daily	2 (milk withhold 0)
Ceftiocyl 50 mg/ml	50 mg ceftiofur/ml	1 ml/16 kg im daily	6
Cevaxel	50 mg ceftiofur/ml	1 ml/16 kg im daily	5
Clamoxyl Ready-to-Use Injection	150 mg amoxicillin/ml	1 ml/20 kg im daily	47
Cobactan 2.5%	25 mg cefquinome/ml	2 ml/25 kg im daily	3
Cobactan 7.5%	75 mg cefquinome/ml	1 ml/25 kg im every 48 h	7
Cyclosol LA	200 mg oxytetracycline/ml	1 ml/10 kg im every 3 days	28
Denagard 200 Solution for Injection	200 mg tiamulin/ml	3 ml/40 kg im daily	14
Depocillin	300 mg procaine benzylpenicillin/ml	1 ml/20 kg im daily	5
Draxxin 100 mg/ml Solution for Injection for Cattle and Pigs	100 mg tulathromycin/ml	1 ml/40 kg im as a single injection	33
Duphacillin	150 mg ampicillin/ml	1 ml/20 kg im daily	18
Duphacycline 10%	100 mg oxytetracycline/ml	1 ml/11–50 kg im daily	20
Duphacycline LA 20% Solution for Injection	200 mg oxytetracycline/ml	1 ml/10 kg im as a single injection	18

Continued

Table A.2. Continued.

Medicine	Active substance	Dose	Meat withhold (days)
Duphamox	150 mg amoxicillin/ml	1 ml/21 kg im daily	16
Duphamox LA	150 mg amoxicillin/ml	1 ml/10 kg im as a single injection	21
Duphapen	300 mg procaine penicillin/ml	1 ml/30 kg im daily	7
Duphapen Fort	300 mg procaine benzylpenicillin/ml	1 ml/15 kg im every 72 h	10
Duphapen+Strep	200 mg procaine benzylpenicillin + 250 mg dihydrostreptomycin per ml	1 ml/25 kg im daily	18
Duphatrim IS Injectable Solution	40 mg trimethoprim + 200 mg sulfadiazine per ml	1 ml/16 kg im daily	20
Eficur	50 mg ceftiofur/ml	1 ml/16 kg im daily	5
Engemycin 10% (DD)	100 mg oxytetracycline/ml	1 ml/12.5 kg im daily or 1 ml/5 kg im every 60 h	14 (with daily dose) 10 (with 60 h dose)
Engemycin 10% Farm Pack	100 mg oxytetracycline/ml	1 ml/12.5 kg im daily or 1 ml/5 kg im every 60 h	14 (with daily dose) 10 (with 60 h dose)
Engemycin LA	200 mg oxytetracycline/ml	1 ml/10 kg im as a single injection	18
Enrocare 5%	50 mg enrofloxacin/ml	1 ml/20 kg im daily (this dose may be doubled when treating salmonellosis and complicated respiratory disease)	10
Enrocare 10%	100 mg enrofloxacin/ml	1 ml/40 kg im daily (this dose may be doubled when treating salmonellosis and complicated respiratory disease)	10
Enroxil Solution for Injection 50 mg/ml for Calves, Pigs and Dogs	50 mg enrofloxacin/ml	1 ml/20 kg im daily (this dose may be doubled when treating salmonellosis and complicated respiratory disease)	10
Enroxil Solution for Injection 100 mg/ml for Calves and Pigs	100 mg enrofloxacin/ml	1 ml/40 kg im daily (this dose may be doubled when treating salmonellosis and complicated respiratory disease)	10
Excenel RTU 50 mg/ml Suspension for Injection for Pigs and Cattle	50 mg ceftiofur/ml	1 ml/16 kg im daily	5
Excenel Sterile Powder for Solution for Injection	50 mg ceftiofur/ml	1 ml/16 kg im daily	2
Fenflor 300 mg/ml Solution for Injection for Pigs	300 mg florfenicol/ml	1 ml/20 kg im every 48 h	18

Continued

Table A.2. Continued.

Medicine	Active substance	Dose	Meat withhold (days)
Fenoflox 50 mg/ml Injection	50 mg enrofloxacin/ml	1 ml/20 kg im daily (this dose may be doubled when treating complicated respiratory disease)	10
Fenoflox 100 mg/ml Injection	100 mg enrofloxacin/ml	1 ml/40 kg im daily (this dose may be doubled when treating complicated respiratory disease)	10
Florkem	300 mg florfenicol/ml	1 ml/20 kg im every 48 h	18
Fosfomycin	This antibiotic is not licensed for use in pigs in the UK. However in other countries it has been found to be a useful antibiotic in respiratory disease	The dose of calcium fosfomycin is 30 mg/kg	42
Intradine	308.9 mg sulfadimidine/ml	1 ml/1.5 kg sc initially followed by 1 ml/3 kg daily	28
Kefloril 300 mg/ml	300 mg florfenicol/ml	1 ml/20 kg im every 48 h	18
Lincocin Sterile Solution	100 mg lincomycin/ml	1 ml/9–22 kg im daily	3
Lincojet 10%	100 mg lincomycin/ml	1 ml/9–22 kg im daily	3
Marbiflox 100 mg/ml Solution for Cattle and Pigs	100 mg marbofloxacin/ml	1 ml/50 kg im daily for 3 days	4
Marbocyl 2% Solution for Injection	2 mg marbofloxacin/ml	1 ml/10 kg im daily	2
Marbocyl 10% Solution for Injection	10 mg marbofloxacin/ml	1 ml/50 kg im daily	2
Marbox 100 mg/ml Solution for Injection for Cattle and Pigs	100 mg marbofloxacin/ml	1 ml/50 kg im daily for 3 days	4
Naxcel 100 mg/ml Suspension for Injection for Pigs	100 mg ceftiofur/ml	1 ml/20 kg im as a single injection	71
Neopen	100 mg neomycin + 200 mg procaine benzylpenicillin per ml	1 ml/20 kg im daily	60
Norobrittin 15%	150 mg ampicillin/ml	1 ml/20 kg im daily	18
Norocillin 30%	300 mg procaine penicillin/ml	1 ml/30 kg im daily	7
Norodine 24	200 mg sulfadiazine + 40 mg trimethoprim per ml	1 ml/16 kg im daily	20
Norotyl LA 15%	150 mg tylosin/ml	1 ml/7.5 kg im as a single injection	7
Nuflor Swine 300 mg/ml Solution for Injection	300 mg florfenicol/ml	1 ml/20 kg im every 48 h	18
Oxycare 10%	100 mg oxytetracycline/ml	1 ml/11–50 kg im daily	20
Oxycare 20% LA	200 mg oxytetracycline/ml	1 ml/10 kg im as a single injection	18

Continued

Table A.2. Continued.

Medicine	Active substance	Dose	Meat withhold (days)
Oxytetrin 20 LA	200 mg oxytetracycline/ml	1 ml/10 kg im as a single injection	70
Pen & Strep	200 mg procaine penicillin + 250 mg dihydrostreptomycin per ml	1 ml/25 kg im daily	18
Penacare	300 mg procaine benzylpenicillin/ml	1 ml/30 kg im daily	7
Powerflox 50 mg/ml Injection	50 mg enrofloxacin/ml	1 ml/20 kg im daily (this rate may be doubled when treating complicated respiratory disease)	10
Powerflox 100 mg/ml Injection	100 mg enrofloxacin/ml	1 ml/40 kg im daily (this rate may be doubled when treating complicated respiratory disease)	10
Readycef Injection	50 mg ceftiofur/ml	1 ml/16 kg im daily	5
Selectan	300 mg florfenicol/ml	1 ml/20 kg im every 48 h	18
Streptacare	200 mg procaine penicillin + 250 mg dihydrostreptomycin per ml	1 ml/25 kg im daily	18
Synulox Ready-To-Use Suspension for Injection	35 mg clavulanic acid + 140 mg amoxicillin per ml	1 ml/20 kg im daily	31
Terramycin Q-100 mg/ml Solution for Injection	100 mg oxytetracycline/ml	1 ml/10 kg im daily	21
Terramycin/LA 200 mg/ml Solution for Injection	200 mg oxytetracycline/ml	1 ml/10 kg im as a single injection	36
Tiamutin 200 Injection	200 mg tiamulin/ml	3 ml/40 kg im daily	14
Tribrissen Injection 48%	80 mg trimethoprim + 80 mg sulfadiazine per ml	1 ml/32 kg im daily	28
Trimacare 24% Injection	40 mg trimethoprim + 200 mg sulfadiazine per ml	1 ml/16 kg im daily	20
Trinacol Injection Solution for Injection	40 mg trimethoprim + 200 mg sulfadiazine per ml	1 ml/16 kg im daily	20
Tylan 200	200 mg tylosin/ml	1 ml/20–100 kg im daily	9
Tyluvet 20% w/v, Solution for Injection	200 mg tylosin/ml	1 ml/20 kg im daily	46
Ultrapen LA	300 mg procaine benzylpenicillin/ml	1 ml/15 kg im as a single injection	10
Vetmulin 162 mg/ml Solution for Injection for Pigs	162 mg tiamulin/ml	1 ml/20 kg im daily	5

Table A.3. Antimicrobials (oral products to be used in the feed or drinking water).

Medicine	Active substance	Dose	Meat withhold (days)
Aivlosin 625 mg/g Granules for Use in Drinking Water	8.5 mg tylvalosin/g	2.125 mg/kg orally in feed for 7 days for treatment of enzootic pneumonia; 4.25 mg/kg orally in feed for 7 days for treatment of porcine proliferative enteropathy (PE) and swine dysentery	2
Amoxinsol 50	50% w/w amoxicillin trihydrate	20 mg/kg in drinking water for 5 days	2
Apralan Soluble Powder	1 g apramycin/sachet or 50 g apramycin/ 220 ml powder	7.5–12.5 mg/kg in drinking water daily for 7 days	14
Chlorsol	50% w/w chlortetracycline	20 mg/kg in drinking water for 5 days	6
Coliscour Solution	2 MIU colistin/ml	0.25 ml/10 kg orally direct into the mouth or in drinking water	1
Denagard 12.5% Oral Solution	125 mg tiamulin/ml	8.8 mg/kg daily in drinking water for 3–5 days	2
HydroDoxx	500 mg doxycycline/g	10 mg doxycycline/kg in drinking water for 5 days	6
Linco-Spectin 100 Soluble Powder	33.3 g lincomycin + 66.7 g spectinomycin per pack	10 mg/kg in drinking water for 7 days	0
Lincocin Soluble Powder	400 g lincomycin/g	4.5 mg/kg in drinking water for a minimum of 5 days	0
Nuflor Drinking Water Concentrate for Swine	23 mg florfenicol/ml	10 mg/kg in drinking water for 5 days	20
Octacillin 697 mg/g Powder for Use in Pigs	697 mg amoxicillin/g	14 mg/kg in drinking water for 3–5 days	2
Pharmasin 100% w/w Water Soluble Granules	110 g tylosin/pot	20 mg/kg for enzootic pneumonia; 5–10 mg/kg for ileitis or porcine intestinal adenomatosis complex (PIA)	1
Pulmodox Granules for Oral Solution	500 mg doxycycline/g	12.5 mg/kg in drinking water for 4 days	4
Selectan Oral	23 mg florfenicol/g	10 mg/kg daily for 5 days	20
Soludox 500 mg/g Water Soluble Powder for Pigs	500 mg doxycycline/g	20 mg/kg in drinking water for 5 days	4
Soludox 500 mg/g Water Soluble Powder for Pigs and Chickens	500 mg doxycycline/g	20 mg/kg in drinking water for 5 days	4
Stabox 50% Oral Soluble Powder for Pigs	500 mg amoxicillin/g	20 mg/kg in liquid feed for 5 days	14
Terramycin Soluble Powder Concentrated 20%	200 g oxytetracycline/kg	10–30 mg/kg in drinking water daily for 3–5 days	7
Tetsol 800	800 g tetracycline hydrochloride/kg	40 mg/kg in drinking water for 5 days	6
Tiamutin 12.5% Solution	125 mg tiamulin/ml	8.8 mg/kg daily in drinking water for 3–5 days	2
Tiamvet 12.5% Solution	125 mg tiamulin/ml	8.8 mg/kg daily in drinking water for 3–5 days	2

Continued

Table A.3. Continued.

Medicine	Active substance	Dose	Meat withhold (days)
Tilmovet 100 mg/g Granules for Pigs	100 mg tilmicosin/g	160 mg/kg daily mixed in individual feed for 15 days	21
Tilmovet 250 mg/ml Concentrate for Oral Solution	250 mg tilmicosin/ml	6–8 ml/100 kg in water daily for 5 days	14
Tylan Soluble	100 g tylosine tartrate/ bottle	25 mg/kg in drinking water for 3–10 days	0
Vetmulin 125 mg/ml Oral Solution	125 mg tiamulin/ml	7 ml/100 kg daily for 5 days for the treatment of swine dysentery; 12–16 ml/110 kg daily for 5 days for the treatment of enzootic pneumonia	5
Vetmulin 450 mg/g Granules for Use in Drinking Water for Pigs	450 mg tiamulin hydrogen fumarate/g	8.8 mg/kg daily for 5 days to treat swine dysentery; 15–20 mg/kg daily for 5 days to treat enzootic pneumonia	5

Table A.4. Antimicrobials (oral products to be given directly by mouth).

Medicine	Active substance	Dose	Meat withhold (days)
Baycox 50 mg/ml Oral Suspension for Piglets, Calves and Lambs	50 mg toltrazuril/ml	0.4 ml/kg once orally	28
Baytril Piglet Doser 0.5% Oral Solution	5 mg enrofloxacin/ml	1 ml once daily orally to piglets under 3 kg daily; 3 ml once daily orally to piglets between 3 and 10 kg	10
Cevazuril 50 mg/ml Oral Suspension	50 mg toltrazuril/ml	0.4 ml/kg once orally	28
Coliscour Solution	2 MIU colistin/ml	0.25 ml/10 kg orally direct into the mouth or in drinking water	1
Spectam Scour Halt	50 mg spectinomycin/ml	1 ml orally twice daily for 3–5 days for piglets under 4.5 kg (the dose should be doubled for heavier piglets)	28
Tratol 50 mg/ml Oral Suspension for Pigs	50 mg toltrazuril/ml	0.4 ml/kg orally once at 3–5 days of age	77

Table A.5. Antimicrobials (topical products).

Medicine	Active substance	Meat withhold (days)
Alamycin Aerosol	Oxytetracycline	0 (meat and milk)
Cyclo Spray	Chlortetracycline	0
Engemycin Spray 3.84% w/w	Oxytetracycline	0
Oxycare Spray	Oxytetracycline	0
Tetcin Aerosol	Oxytetracycline	0

Cardiovascular and respiratory preparations

These are rarely used in commercial pig practice. They may have a place in the treatment of pet pigs. Medicines are listed in Table A.6.

Dietary supplements and fluid metabolites

These are particularly useful for smallholder pigs where feeding practices may not be optimum. Iron injections are rarely necessary in any outdoor pigs. However they are vital for piglets born inside. Medicines are listed in Table A.7.

Table A.6. Cardiovascular and respiratory preparations (injectable and oral).

Medicine	Active substance	Dose	Meat withhold (days)
Bisolvon Injection	3 mg bromhexine/ml	7–17 ml/100 kg im daily	28
Bisolvon Powder	10 mg bromohexine/g	2–5 g/100 kg in drinking water daily	0

Table A.7. Dietary supplements and fluid metabolites (injectable and oral).

Medicine	Active substance	Dose	Meat withhold (days)
Anvit 4BC Injection	35 mg thiamin + 0.5 mg riboflavin + 7 mg pyridoxine + 23 mg nicotinamide + 70 mg ascorbic acid per ml	5–10 ml im, iv or sc per pig daily	0
Duphafral Multivitamin 9	15,000 IU retinol + 25 µg cholecalciferol + 20 mg α-tocopheryl acetate + 10 mg thiamin + 5 mg riboflavin + 3 mg pyridoxine + 35 mg nicotinamide + 25 mg dexpanthenol per ml	5–10 ml im or sc per pig; 2–5 ml per weaner	28
Duphalyte	A combination of B-complex vitamins, electrolytes, amino acids and dextrose	100 ml/50 kg iv for adults; 30 ml/5 kg for younger pigs (this may be followed up by sc injections)	0
Effydral Effervescent Tablet	2.34 g sodium chloride + 1.12 g potassium chloride + 6.72 g sodium bicarbonate + 3.84 g citric acid + 32.44 g lactose + 2.25 g glycine per tablet	1 tablet in 1 litre of water, give ad lib to pigs	0
Forgastrin Oral Powder	73% attapulgite–27% bone charcoal	6–10 g thrice daily for pigs as a drench with a little water or in a little food; mix 10 g in 60 ml of water and give 5 ml daily to piglets	0
Gleptosil Injection	200 mg gleptoferron iron/ml	1 ml per piglet im once	0
Intravit 12	0.5 g cyanobalamin/ml	0.5–1.5 ml im or sc per pig	0
Lectade Powder for Oral Solution	Sachet A: 6.18 g glycine + 0.48 g citric acid + 0.12 g potassium citrate + 4.08 g potassium dihydrogen phosphate + 8.58 g sodium chloride. Sachet B: 44.61 g glucose	Add both sachets to 2 litres of water; solution should be readily available to young pigs	0
Liquid Life-Aid	Concentrated aqueous solution for dilution with 11.5 times its own volume of water	200–300 ml per piglet orally per day; 1 litre per weaned pig daily	0
Multivitamin Injection	15,000 IU vitamin A + 25 µg vitamin D + 20 mg vitamin E + 10 mg vitamin B_1 + 5 mg vitamin B_2 + 3 mg vitamin B_6 + 35 mg nicotinamide + 25 mg dexpanthenol + 25 µg vitamin B_{12} per ml	5–10 ml per adult (2 – 5 ml per weaner; 0.5–2 ml per piglet) im or sc, repeated in 10–14 days	28
Vitesel	68 mg α-tocopheryl acetate + 1.5 mg potassium selenate per ml	1 ml/25 kg im to piglets to be repeated in 2–4 weeks	0

Antiparasitic preparations

Commercial pigs are likely to be treated on a regular basis by in-feed parasiticides. The medications described in Table A.8 are very useful in smallholder and pet pigs.

Other medicines

These medicines are included in Table A.9 for completeness. Their usage is described in the relevant chapters.

Medicines Useful in Pigs not Licensed for Pigs but Licensed for Other Species

It should be remembered that as these medicines are not licensed for pigs, they have an automatic 28-day meat withhold. Preparations are listed in Table A.10.

Table A.8. Antiparasitic preparations (injectable and oral).

Medicine	Active substance	Dose	Meat withhold (days)
Alstomec	10 mg ivermectins/ml	1 ml/33 kg sc	28
Animec Injection	10 mg ivermectins/ml	1 ml/33 kg sc	28
Dectomax 10 mg/ml Solution for Injection for Pigs	10 mg doramectin/ml	1 ml/33 kg im	56
Flubenol 5% w/w Oral Powder for Pigs	50 mg flubendazole/g	1 g/10 kg in feed as a single dose	7
Ivomec Injection for Pigs	10 mg ivermectins/ml	1 ml/33 kg sc	19
Noromectin Multi Injection	10 mg ivermectins/ml	1 ml/33 kg sc	28
Panacur 1.5% Pellets	15 mg fenbendazole/g	5 g/15 kg in feed	3
Panomec Injection for Cattle, Sheep and Pigs	10 mg ivermectins/ml	1 ml/33 kg sc	19
Qualimec 10 mg/ml Solution for Injections	10 mg ivermectins/ml	1 ml/33 kg sc	28
Solubenol 100 mg/g Oral Emulsion	100 mg flubendazole/g	1 g/100 kg daily in water for 5 days	4
Virbamec Injectable Solution for Cattle, Swine and Sheep	10 mg ivermectins/ml	1 ml/33 kg sc	28

Table A.9. Other medicines.

Medicine	Active substance	Dose	Meat withhold (days)
Altresyn	4 mg altrenogest/ml	5 ml to be given orally to gilts for 18 consecutive days	24
Cyclix Porcine	0.0875 mg cloprostenol sodium/ml	2 ml as a single injection per sow as a deep im injection	2
Enzaprost	5 mg dinoprost/ml	2 ml per pig im	2
Gestavet 600	400 IU serum gonadotrophin + 200 IU chorionic gonadotrophin per 5 ml dose	To be given as im injection	??
Lethobarb	20% w/v pentobarbital sodium	0.7 ml/kg iv	Not to be used in animals intended for human and animal consumption
Lutalyse 5 mg/ml Solution for Injection	5 mg dinoprost/ml	2 ml per sow im	1

Continued

Table A.9. Continued.

Medicine	Active substance	Dose	Meat withhold (days)
Maprelin 75 µg/ml	75 µg perforelin/ml	0.5 ml per primiparous sow im; 2 ml per pluriparous sow im after weaning off the piglets; 2 ml per gilt 48 h after the termination of the medication for inhibition of the cycle	0
Monzaldon 100 mg/ml Solution for Injection	100 mg vetrabutine hydrochloride/ml	2–4 ml per sow im as a single injection	28
Oxytocin-S	10 IU oxytocin/ml	0.2–1 ml im as a single dose	0
Pentobarbital for Euthanasia 20% Solution for Injection	20% w/v pentobarbital sodium	0.7 ml/kg iv	Not to be used in animals intended for human and animal consumption
PG 600	400 IU serum gonadotrophin + 200 IU chorionic gonadotrophin per 5 ml dose	To be given as im injection	0
Planate	0.0875 mg cloprostenol sodium/ml	2 ml as a single injection per sow as a deep im injection	2
PMSG-INTERVET 5000 IU Powder and Solvent for Solution for Injections	5000 IU serum gonadotrophin (PMSG) supplied together with solvent, which when reconstituted gives a solution containing 200 IU PMSG/ml	5 ml to be given im or sc as a single injection per sow	0
Prosolvin Solution for Injection	7.5 mg luprostiol/ml	1 ml as a single injection per sow im	4
Receptal 0.004 mg/ml Solution for Injection	0.004 mg buserelen/ml	2.5 ml per pig im or iv, with AI 30–33 h later	0
Regumate Porcine	0.4% w/v altrenogest	Gilts should be given 5 ml daily for 18 consecutive days orally; sows should be given 5 ml daily for 3 consecutive days	24
Reprocine	0.07 mg carbetocin/ml	1.5–3 ml per sow im or iv (can be repeated in 48 h)	0
Sterilised Water for Injection BP			0
Stresnil 40 mg/ml Solution for Injection for Pigs	40 mg azaperone/ml	0.5–1 ml/20 kg im	10
Virbagest 4 mg/ml Oral Solution for Pigs	4 mg altrenogest/ml	5 ml to be given orally to gilts for 18 consecutive days	24
Water for Injection			0

Table A.10. Medicines useful in pigs not licensed for pigs but licensed for other species.

Medicine	Active substance	Dose	Meat withhold (days)
Buscopan Composition	4 mg butylsopolamine bromide + 500 mg metamizole per ml	1 ml/10 kg im (this product may have a use in treating bowel obstruction and blockage of the urethra or ureters)	28

Glossary

___

Abortion – premature birth of young.

Active immunity – immunity obtained by the pig from either natural infection or vaccination.

Acute – a disease with a sudden onset.

Aetiology – cause of a disease.

Agalactia – lack of milk.

Annual – a plant which grows from seed, flowers and dies within a year.

Anorexia – not eating.

Anthelmintics – drugs that expel parasitic worms from the body, generally by paralysing or starving them.

Antigen – a molecule or part of a molecule that is recognized by components of the host immune system.

Arthrogryposis –wrongly developed joints.

Ataxia – difficulty with stable movement.

Atresia ani – absence of an anus.

Autosomal chromosome – a non-sex chromosome.

Awn – a bristle or hair-like appendage to a fruit or to a glume, as in barley and some other grasses.

Bacteraemia – bacteria in the blood.

Biennial – a plant which flowers and dies in the second year after growing from a seed.

Bradycardia – decrease in heart rate.

Bronchitis – inflammation of the bronchi.

Bruxism – grinding of teeth.

Bursitis – inflammation of a bursa (a fluid-filled sack protecting a tendon).

Calculi – stones formed in the urinary system.

Cerebral – relating to the cerebrum, the largest part of the brain.

Cestodes – parasitic flatworms, commonly called tapeworms, which usually live in the digestive tract of vertebrates as adults and in the bodies of various intermediate hosts as juvenile stages.

Chronic – a disease with a slow onset.

Colitis – inflammation of the colon; often used to describe an inflammation of the large intestine.

Colostrum – the milk supplied by the mother for the first two days after the young have been born. It supplies vital antibodies to disease to the young, giving them passive immunity.

Coma – profound unconsciousness from which the patient cannot be roused.

Congestion – the presence of an abnormal amount of blood in an organ or part.

Contusions – bruises.

Convulsion – a violent involuntary contraction of muscles.

Coritis – inflammation of the corium (the point where the skin joins the hoof).

Corm – underground bulbous root.

Cystitis – inflammation of the bladder.

Deciduous plants – Those which shed all their leaves annually.

Dermatitis – an inflammation of the dermis (all of the skin structures).

Detoxicate – to render a poison harmless.

Distension – the filling of a hollow organ to more than its usual capacity.

Diuresis – excessive urination.

DNA fingerprinting – much like the fingerprint used in human identification, but done with unique DNA characters for each individual animal. Utilizes PCR to replicate small samples.

Dysentery – an illness characterized by diarrhoea with blood in the faeces.

Dysphagia – difficulty in swallowing.

Dyspnoea – difficulty in breathing.

Dystocia – difficulty at parturition.

Egg reappearance period – the time taken (usually expressed in weeks) for eggs to reappear in faeces after anthelmintic treatment. Usually this is described for drug-sensitive worm populations at the time of product licensing.

ELISA – a technique used primarily in immunology to detect the presence of an antibody or an antigen in a sample. Basically, an unknown amount of antigen is bound to the surface of a plastic well; then a specific antibody is added and, if specific, will bind the antigen. This antibody is linked to an enzyme or is detected by incubation with a second antibody that is linked to an enzyme. In the final step a substance is added that the enzyme can convert to some detectable signal (usually a colour change which is detectable by a spectrophotometer).

Emaciation – excessive body wasting.

Emesis – vomiting.

Emetic – a substance which causes vomiting.

Encephalitis – an inflammation of the brain in general.

Encephalomyelitis – an inflammation of the myelin, i.e. the white part of the brain.

Endocarditis – an inflammation of the endocardium, i.e. the inside of the heart, particularly the heart valves.

Enteritis – an inflammation of the intestine.

Enteropathy – a pathological change to the intestine.

Epidemiology – the study of factors affecting the health of populations and often how diseases are transmitted.

Epiphysiolysis – a weakening of the cartilage of a joint, particularly as it lifts off the bone tissue.

Epistaxis – bleeding down the nose.

Farrowing – the process of a pig giving birth.

Foetid – malodorous.

Genome – an organism's entire hereditary information, encoded either in DNA or, for some types of virus, in RNA. The genome includes the genes that code the proteins and non-coding sequences of the DNA.

Genotype – the inherited instructions organisms carry in their genetic code.

Gilt – female pig yet to have had piglets; may be unserved or in-pig.

Granules – small grains.

Haematuria – blood in the urine.

Haemolytic – a substance which causes breakdown of red blood cells.

Helminths – a group of eukaryotic parasites that live inside their host. They are worm-like and live and feed off animals.

Hepatitis – inflammation of the liver.

Herbaceous perennials – plants in which the greater part dies after flowering, leaving only the rootstock to produce next year's growth.

Herd – the collective word for a group of pigs.

Hernia – may be a deficiency of abdominal muscles as in umbilical and inguinal hernias, or damage to the abdominal muscles as in a rupture caused by trauma.

Hydrops allantois – an excess of allantoic fluid formed around the fetus.

Hypoglycaemia – a low blood glucose.

Iatrogenic – resulting from treatment.

Ileitis – an inflammation of the ileum (the nearest small intestine to the large intestine).

Ileus – failure of peristalsis.

Inappetence – not eager to eat (this is not as severe as anorexia).

Inco-ordination – not able to place the legs correctly (this is not as severe as ataxia).

Indigenous – native of the country in which it was produced.

In-pig – pregnant pig.

Intussusception – when a part of the small or large intestine becomes inverted into itself.

In extremis – at the point of death.

In vitro – in the test-tube.

In vivo – in the living body.

Jaundice – a disease in which bile pigments stain the mucous membranes.

Laminitis – an inflammation of the laminae (the tissue that actually connects the wall of the hoof to the pedal bone).

Larvae – juvenile forms that many animals undergo before the mature adult stage. Larvae are frequently adapted to environments different from those adult stages live in.

Linear leaves – those that are long and narrow.

Luer fitting – this is the standard EU fitting for a needle and syringe (record fitting used to be used in the UK).

Lumen – the inner space of a tubular structure, such as the intestine.

Lymphadenopathy – a swelling of the lymph system, mainly the lymph nodes.

Marker – a short tandem repeat (STR) that may be used to aid in the identification of a trait.

Mediastinum – space in the chest between the lungs.

Melaena – dark tarry faeces indicating bleeding high in the intestinal tract.

Meningitis – an inflammation of the covering of the brain.

Metritis – inflammation of the uterus.

Micturition – the passing of urine.

Mutations – alterations in DNA sequence in a genome that spontaneously occur during meiosis or DNA replication or are caused by factors such as by radiation, viruses or chemicals. Mutations can have no effect or they can alter the product of a gene from functioning properly, if at all.

Myelopathy – a pathological change in the white areas of the brain.

Myiasis – fly strike.

Myoglobinuria – breakdown products from the muscles appearing in the urine.

Narcosis – sleep induced by a drug or poison.

Nematodes – roundworms, one of the most diverse phyla of all animals.

Nephritis – an inflammation of the kidney.

Nodule – a small round lump.

Nucleotide – the building blocks of DNA; composed of deoxyribose sugars, a phosphate and one of four nitrogenous bases.

Nystagmus – a specific neurological sign seen in the eye. The eye moves slowly laterally and then flicks back medially.

Oedema – fluid in tissues.

Opisthotonous – a neurological sign when the head and spine are bent backwards.

Orchitis – inflammation of the testicle.
Osteochondritis – inflammation of bone and cartilage.
Osteochondrosis – damage to bone and cartilage.
Osteomalacia – thin weak bones lacking in calcium.
Paracentesis – the technique of puncturing a body cavity.
Parakeratosis – an overproduction of keratin in the skin, i.e. a thickening.
Parenteral – a medicine given to the whole body.
Paresis – a lack of ability to move the body or a specific limb.
Parturition – the act of giving birth.
Passive immunity – immunity acquired by young animals from drinking colostrum.
Pathogenicity – the ability of a pathogen to produce signs of disease in an organism.
Pathognomonic – a single specific single sign of a disease.
PCR – a technique to amplify a single or a few copies of a piece of DNA by several orders
   of magnitude, generating thousands to millions of copies of a particular sequence. PCR
   relies on cycles of repeated heating and cooling of DNA and enzymatic replication of DNA.
   Primers (short DNA fragments) containing sequences complementary to the target region
   along with a DNA polymerase (after which the method is named) are key components to
   enable selective and repeated amplification. As PCR progresses, DNA generated is used
   as a template for replication, setting in motion a chain reaction in which the template is
   exponentially amplified.
Peracute – a disease with an extremely rapid onset.
Pericarditis – an inflammation of the outside of the heart.
Peritonitis – an inflammation of the peritoneum, the covering of all the organs in the abdomen.
Petechia – small haemorrhages.
Phenotype – any observable characteristic or trait of an organism such as its morphology,
   development, biochemical or physiological properties, or behaviour. Phenotypes result
   from the expression of an organism's genes as well as the influence of environmental
   factors and possible interactions between the two.
Pleurisy – an inflammation of the covering of the lungs.
Polyarthritis – inflammation of many joints.
Polyserositis – an inflammation of all the serous surfaces in the body, e.g. the peritoneum,
   the pleura, the pericardium, etc.
Premix – medicine available in a concentrated form to be added to food.
Prepatent period – the time between an egg of a nematode being swallowed by the pig and
   the time it has become an adult and eggs appear in the faeces.
Primer – several thousand copies of short sequences of DNA that are complementary to part
   of the DNA to be sequenced.
Prolapse – an evagination of an organ.
Proteomics – the study of proteins in feed.
Pruritis – irritation of the skin.
Purgative – a strong laxative.
Pyelonephritis – pus in the kidneys.
Pyrexia – raised rectal temperature.
RAPD PCR (random amplification of polymorphic DNA–PCR) – a specific diagnostic test.
Recumbency – unable to get up.
Retroversion – when the bladder comes through the urethra.
Rhinitis – inflammation of the nose.
RT-PCR (reverse transcriptase PCR) – a specific diagnostic test.
Sclerosis – hardening of a tissue.
Seborrhoea – a skin condition where there is excess sebum, i.e. oily secretion.
Septicaemia – pathogenic bacteria in the blood.
Slough – dead tissue which drops away from living tissue.

Spasm – involuntary contraction of a muscle.

Stomatitis – inflammation of the mouth and gums.

STR (short tandem repeats) – sections of DNA arranged in back-to-back repetition.

Stricture – a narrowing of a tubular organ.

Subacute – a disease with a relatively rapid onset.

Subclinical – when the symptoms are not evident.

Syndrome – a group of symptoms.

Tachycardia – increased heart rate.

Tenesmus – straining to pass urine or faeces.

Torpid – sluggish.

Tourniquet – an appliance for temporary stoppage of the circulation in a limb.

Ubiquitous – everywhere.

Udder – mammary gland.

Ureter – the tube connecting the kidney to the bladder.

Urethra – the tube leading from the bladder to outside.

Urethritis – inflammation of the urethra.

Urolithiasis – the formation of stones in the urinary system.

Uticaria – an acute inflammatory reaction of the skin.

Vaginitis – inflammation of the vagina.

Vagus – tenth cranial nerve.

Venereal disease – a disease spread by coitus.

Vesicle – a collection of fluid in the surface layers of the skin or of a mucous membrane.

Viraemia – virus particles in the blood.

Volatile – a substance which evaporates rapidly.

Volvulus – a twist of the intestine.

Zoonosis – disease communicable between animals and man.

References

Blank, R., Muller-Siegwardt, B. and Wolffram, S. (2010) Sanguinarine does not influence availability or metabolism of tryptophan in pigs. *Livestock Science* 134, 24–26.

Brightman, C. (2012) Rabies: an acute viral infection. *Trends in Urology & Men's Health* 1, 31–33.

Brown, P. (2012) Vaccines: perception and reality. *Pig & Poultry Marketing* Winter 2012 issue, 42.

Carr, J. and Smith, J. (2013) Storage and safe use of medicines on farm. *In Practice* 35, 36–42.

Chaturvedi, M.M., Kumar, A., Darnay, B.G., Chainy, G.B.N., Agarwal, S. and Aggarwal, B.B. (1997) Sanguinarine (pseudochelerythine) is a potent inhibitor of NF-κB activation, IκBκ phosphorylation, and degradation. *Journal of Biological Chemistry* 271, 30129–30134.

Coggins, L. (1968) A modified haemadsorption-inhibition test for African swine fever virus. *Bulletin of Epizootic Diseases of Africa* 16, 61–64.

Corona, E.B., Spiru, D., Li, D. and McOrist, S. (2012) Evaluations of limiting amino acid uptake in finisher pigs dosed orally with sanguinarine alkaloids. *The Pig Journal* 67, 39–42.

Del Pozo Sacristan, R., Rodriguez, A.L., Sierens, A., Maes, D.G.D., Vranckx, K., Boyen, F., Haesebrouck, F. and Dereu, A. (2012) Efficacy of in-feed medication with chlortetracycline in a farrow-to-finish herd against a clinical outbreak of respiratory disease in fattening pigs. *Veterinary Record* 171, 645.

Drsata, J., Ulrichoa, J. and Walterova, D. (1996) Sanguinarine and chelerythrine as inhibitors of aromatic amino acid decarboxylase. *Journal of Enzyme Inhibition and Medicinal Chemistry* 10, 231–237.

Groenen, M.A.M., Archibald, A.L., Uenishi, H. and Tuggle, C.K. (2012) Pig 'reference genome' could provide benefits for agriculture and medicine. *Nature* 491, 393–398.

Guiterrez, A.M., Nobauer, K., Soler, L., Razzazi-Fazeli, E., Gemeiner, M., Ceron, J.J. and Miller, I. (2012) Potential markers for systemic disease in the saliva of pigs. *Veterinary Immunology and Pathology* 151, 73–82.

Harley, S., More, S.J., O'Connell, N.E., Hanlon, A., Teixeira, D. and Boyle, L. (2012) Evaluating the prevalence of tail-biting and carcase condemnations in slaughter pigs in Republic and Northern Ireland, and the potential of abattoir meat inspection as a welfare surveillance tool. *Veterinary Record* 171, 621.

Jackson, P.G.G. and Cockcroft, P.D. (eds) (2007) Carbon monoxide poisoning: anoxia due to carboxyhaemoglobin in piglets. In: *Handbook of Pig Medicine*. Saunders Elsevier, Philadelphia, Pennsylvania, p. 154.

Lambooij, E. (2012) Pig welfare and what you can tell from the carcase. *Veterinary Record* 171, 619–620.

Marino, M., Maifreni, M., Moret, S. and Ronodinini, N. (2000) The capacity of Enterobacteriaceae species to produce biogenic amines in cheese. *Letters in Applied Microbiology* 31, 169–173.

Millar, M. and Stack, J. (2012) Brucellosis – what every practitioner should know. *In Practice* 34, 532–539.

Nathues, H., Woeste, H., Doehring, S., Fahrion, A.S., Doherr, M.G. and grosse Beilage, E. (2012) Detection of *Mycoplasma hyopneumoniae* in nasal swabs sampled from pig farmers. *Veterinary Record* 170, 623.

Niven, S.J., Beal, J.D. and Brooks, P.H. (2006) The effect of controlled fermentation on the fate of synthetic lysine in liquid diets for pigs. *Animal Feed Science and Technology* 129, 304–313.

Normand, V., Perrin, H., Laval, A., Auvigne, V. and Robert, N. (2012) Anaemia in the sow: a cohort study to assess factors with an impact on haemoglobin concentration, and the influence of haemoglobin concentration on the reproductive performance. *Veterinary Record* 171, 350.

Novosel, D., Cubric-Curik, V., Jungic, A. and Lipej, Z. (2012) Presence of Torque teno suis virus in porcine circovirus type 2-associated disease in Croatia. *Veterinary Record* 171, 529.

O'Neill, K.C., Hemann, M., Gimenez-Lirola, L.G., Halbur, P.G. and Opriessnig, T. (2012) Vaccination of sows reduces the prevalence of PCV-2 viraemia in their piglets under field conditions. *Veterinary Record* 171, 425.

Santos, M.H.S. (1998) Amino acid decarboxylase capability of micro-organisms isolated in Spanish fermented meat products. *International Journal of Food Microbiology* 39, 227–230.

Sims, L. (2012) Keeping track of swine influenza virus. *Veterinary Record* 171, 269–270.

Smith, G.J., Vijaykrishna, D., Bahl, J., Lycett, S.J., Worobey, M., Pybus, O.G., Ma, S.K., Cheung, C.L., Raghwani, J., Bhatt, S., Peiris, J.S., Guan, Y. and Rambaut, A. (2009) Origins and evolutionary genomics of the 2009 swine origin H1N1 influenza A epidemic. *Nature* 459, 1122–1125.

Stephano, H.A., Gay, G.M. and Ramirez, T.C. (1988) Encephalomyelitis, reproductive failure and corneal opacity (blue eye) in pigs, associated with a new paramyovirus infection. *Veterinary Record* 122, 6–10.

Index